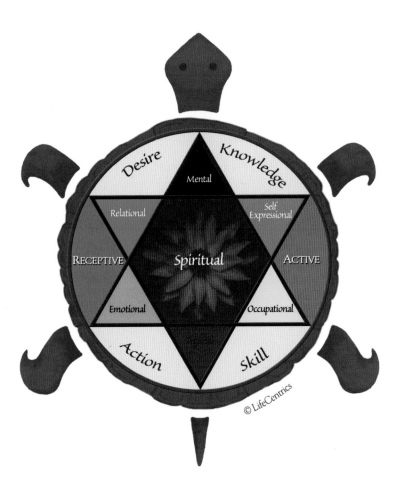

© LifeCentrics

The Art of Self-Health
A Model for Integrative Wellness

The Art of
SELF-HEALTH

Creating Total Well-Being from the Inside Out

Carol LaRue

LifeCentrics

Dedicated to
Courtney Renee Lett,
whose spirit of love
guides and inspires me
to be love.

Published by LifeCentrics, Jay, OK 74346

ISBN 978-0-9835070-0-0

Library of Congress Control Number: 2011914591

Cover design, book design and illustrations by Pamela Hawkins, Indigo Creative Space
Photography by Bill LaRue

Published 2011
Printed in Hong Kong

TABLE OF CONTENTS

FOREWORD

I first met Carol when I attended one of her movement (Nia) classes. I, like so many in our culture, tend to live "in my head" and I knew that I needed some kind of body-centered activity. What I experienced on that first day was a group of women moving and dancing together with such joy and exuberance that I was reduced to tears. Women of all ages, all shapes and sizes and varying levels of physical prowess were being led into a full expression of their individual radiance. Carol guided the class with a free and relaxed manner that invited full participation and absolutely no sense of competition. I began attending classes twice a week, and although my level of fitness certainly improved, there was something even deeper going on. My awareness of my body, and my ability to actually *enjoy* my body were being nurtured. In addition, every class was emotionally healing and richly spiritual. I found that I was able to be more authentic in my daily life—more grounded, more present and more "at home with myself."

Carol walks her talk. She *embodies* the art of self-health. This book is a beautiful expression of who she is, and is a masterful guide for those of us who want to be healthy in mind, body and spirit. Carol's wisdom comes from her heart—and from her personal life experience. She has known great sorrow and profound life changes since I first met her in 2002. She has not merely "survived;" she has transformed adversity into strength and open-hearted generosity.

I have had the privilege of co-facilitating workshops with Carol and have admired her leadership skills and her ability to foster self-discovery and transformation in others. Many men and women are extremely uncomfortable moving their bodies in a group setting. Carol has a gift for enabling even the "shyest of the shy" to move more freely and unselfconsciously and to be at home in their bodies.

One of the most impressive of Carol's skills is her use of the chakra system to integrate mind, body and spirit. This ancient bio-energetic system has become foundational in the practice of current holistic and alternative medicine. As you will see as you read this book, Carol uses the chakras as a map for the journey of personal transformation and offers practical exercises that balance and stimulate the energy of each chakra.

In our culture of stress, anxiety, workaholism and competition, many adults neglect their bodies. The number of people requiring anti-depressant and/or anti-anxiety medication continues to rise. Obesity is an increasing epidemic in our society. Reliance on stimulant substances (such as caffeine) and abuse of stimulant prescription medications are ongoing, serious health risks. This book presents an alternative to our self-destructive lifestyles.

I urge you to read this book. I urge you to *work* this book and recommend it to your friends. It has the power to improve the way you feel about yourself, to enhance your relationships with other people, and to transform the way you live your life.

Lisa Whitlow, M.A., D.Min.

3

It is man's foremost duty to awaken the understanding of the inner Self

and to know his own real inner greatness.

Once he knows his true worth, he can know the worth of others.

Therefore, meditate on your Self, honor and worship your own Self,

kneel to your own Self, and see the Lord who is hidden in your own heart.

SWAMI MUKTANANDA

INTRODUCTION

4

My entire being—body, mind and spirit remembers feeling so good, so connected and so powerful from the inside-out. The memory of that warm, expansive sensation keeps calling me back. Back to my self, where every cell of my body vibrates with light and joy. My heart celebrates remembering my song of inner knowing, inner bliss and inner peace.

AUTHOR'S JOURNAL ENTRY 2006

Many of us have forgotten this "feel good" place, yet it is where we all belong and where we can all feel safe and thrive. Sometimes we can remember and even recreate this feeling of being in balance. Sometimes it must be reborn through present awareness, learning and gathering new resources. Whatever your journey of reconnecting to self, it is a journey worth embarking on.

More years than not, I spent in the darkness of my full radiance. My navigation through life took far more energy than needed because I was not plugged into my true source of energy—my SELF. I was too concerned and busy pleasing others and doing for others. My awakening, which at times came slowly and easily and at times harsh and fast, led me to discover the power of what many have known for ages. Through trial and error, I discovered and experienced age-old wisdom and practices such as mindfulness, yoga and meditation and their practicality for re-creating lightness and joy, everyday—even in the fast-paced world of modern day. While the chaos of our present-day world threatens both our individual balance and our collective global balance, the world is still thirsty for us to reclaim responsibility for our individual health and wellness. As we saturate ourselves in healthful practices, our individual vibrancy returns and the world's thirst for balance is quenched, one individual at a time. While I dream of a world full of energetic, joyful and healthy individuals, I know that I must first be the change I want to see. First, I must remember my SELF.

*It was the late 1950's. We were on a family vacation and celebrating my fifth birthday with my favorite aunt, uncle and cousins in Casper, Wyoming. At five, I couldn't describe my feelings other than, **"I feel good, I am happy and I am loved!"** but I remember that experience, so I know what joy, personal power and love feels like! My aunt made a beautiful and unique blue square-layered birthday cake and I got the exact present that I wished for—plastic high heeled shoes, just my size that went perfectly with any dress-up gig I could imagine. I was having so much fun being prissy, dancing and flaunting my "grown up and pretty self" in the company of my favorite cousins and family. I was on top of the world! Looking back, I still smile big, remembering joy, belonging, love, spirited imagination, free dancing and my "I am the queen!" attitude.*

5

Fast forward 41 years later to 1999. Little did I know that my decision to leave a corporate job to begin a business dedicated to health and wellness education would catapult me into a ten-year journey of self-discovery and self-health. I realize now that the business I started, LifeCentrics, was a divinely-inspired and divinely-timed platform for reconnecting my self to the center of my life. It's true. We teach what we most need to learn.

My journey began in November 1999. I am searching for my self. I lost her somehow. I am burned out on work, a fast-paced life and my 15 year marriage. I want so much to create joy and a feeling of whole health in my life. I've decided to quit smoking, again. I am in the middle of a week-long training intensive on The Nia Technique® and I can't stop crying! My tears of relief and joy are flowing non-stop along with a little bit of fear. I have found that feeling again! I am dancing, and I have come home to myself. I am once again feeling my pleasure, my power and my purpose. Why the fear? Because somehow I know that my life will never be the same. And yet I feel good and I feel strong. I feel like I am connected to and being pulled into something way larger than myself, yet it is my SELF. And it is just the beginning. As I will learn, and am still learning, I may stray from my self again and again, but I can always return, because my home—my place of comfort, ease, belonging, peace, joy and power—is always within my

SELF, so I don't have to go far to find it.

This place on the inside feels like a big comfy chair. It's that place where it doesn't matter what my name is, what kind of work I do, how well I dress or dance, who I am related to, what my dreams are or what my story is. And it *feels good*. It's broken in. It fits just right, because it is where I can completely and authentically be ME, my SELF. We all have a comfy chair. It is the place where we began this life and the place where we will end this life. It is the place where we are always whole, complete, creative and loving. It brings us feelings of pleasure, power and purpose. It is the place within our being where we can relax and not feel lazy, let our imaginations soar and our dreams clarify. It is the place where we can stretch big, dance passionately and walk briskly, while feeling the miracle and the vitality of our body. It is the place where we can snuggle contently with our beloved, knowing that we are loved, and our hearts open freely to love our self and others. It is home. ME today is the same five-year-old ME who felt like she had it all! It is that place within each of us that never really changes.

Rediscovering something that I have always known has been a long and arduous journey. The more I learn, the more I want to learn. My capacity for seeking and learning feels like a deep well that requires continuous replenishment. Fortunately for all of us, this planet has been graced with an abundance of wise teachers and sages. These are our way-showers and our guides who are willing to share their insights, experiences and wisdom through books, films, workshops and inspirational presentations. I see these teachers as tributaries that feed and nurture the streams of consciousness which in turn feed the vast oceanic source of wisdom we all tap into if we choose. Through this vast ocean of knowledge and experience we can satisfy our cravings for meaningful sustenance. I am eternally grateful to these teachers, many of whom I have never met. In many respects I too am a wisdom teacher. My wisdom has been awakened over the years by my everyday life experience, most of it a process of discovery. My wisdom is an everyday wisdom put into practice in everyday practical living. I share this writing humbly, with the awareness that I am a second stage messenger for information that has positively changed my life. I hope that the lessons and experiences that have transformed my everyday approach to living life as healthfully as possible can positively influence your life.

This book is an accumulation of my practical life applications while I searched for personal balance, meaning and fulfillment, often in a chaotic and disruptive world. These lessons have been many and varied—an unexpected teenage pregnancy, failed marriages, reuniting with my birth son after 30 years, my daughter's sudden death, starting and losing businesses, being part of an expansive and supportive community of friends, meeting and marrying the love of my life in middle age, facing down breast cancer, relocating after 30 years to a simpler life in a place of natural wonder—just to name a few! Whew! I am not sure my life is any more chaotic or subject to sudden changes than others, but I like to think of each of the life-defining events in my life as opportunities to bring my SELF and my self-health more clearly into focus. I believe that all experiences are potential paths to self-discovery and opportunities to understand more deeply what we need for personal awareness and expansion. Our life experiences simply allow us to tap into the resiliency of our human spirit! So, here is my humble attempt to deliver everyday, real-life wisdom for everyday energy and well-being. Here is what I *do* know—that we all have the capacity to become more aware of our SELF while influencing our personal energy, health and experiences by the everyday choices we make, specifically by:

- what we eat, how we move and how we rest
- how we feel and process emotions
- how we share our unique gifts and talents
- how we relate
- how we express ourselves
- what we think and how we perceive and interpret events
- how we experience a connection to the divine *and* allow ourselves to BE.

Our lives are creative masterpieces and an everyday work of art, moment by moment. Every moment of every day we make choices that ultimately color the canvas of our lives. Each choice we make contributes to the creation of the whole being. The creation of our masterpieces can be the art of self-destruction, the art of self-stagnation or the art of self-health (healing). Actually, we may have created a bit of each scenario throughout our lives, but we always have a choice. Creating health often begins with un-doing, creating time and space to fill the canvas with a more joyful and healthful expression of our selves. Do-overs are okay. If something isn't working or taking up unnecessary space and time in your life, let it go.

Life is an everyday event. Whether we like it or not it is often filled with the stress of home, the stress of work, personal and professional challenges, loss, fear, frustration, emptiness, illness, sadness, etc. Here enters some early wisdom of the ancient turtle, which we will learn more from in future chapters. *Like the ancient turtle, our resilience to the ups and downs of life depends on our ability to **adapt and change**.* And in order to see and evaluate what our choices are, *just like the turtle, we have to be willing to **stick our necks out*** to explore our options. The good news is that our comfy chair, just like the turtle's protective shell, is not far away! Our comfy chair can be found right NOW, where we are. So we start where we are, and we can always come back, settle in, and see how we feel before taking the next step on this journey to self-health.

This book is intended to be a fluid and dynamic resource tool. Use it as a reference, use it for inspiration and/or use it as a workbook. It is not intended to be directive or to present hard-line rules of healthy living. You are invited to see each section of the book as a color of paint on your palette. You can move freely between chapters, dipping your brush into whatever color you need at the time. *Your life is a work of art* that unfolds naturally. You can't push a river. You can't change the length of time the sun shines each day. What you *can* do is *influence* the experience of your life, each day, by the choices you make every moment. Again, start where you are! This book is not intended to instantaneously wash away life as you know it today, but to provide you with information and choices. It offers simple tools, in natural time, for creating *balance* from *busyness* and *self-health* from *dis-ease*. *(No, this isn't a typo.* **Dis-ease** *implies the lack of ease in living, which can contribute to* **disease** *and illness)*. We all have the ability to choose self-health everyday.

Like many, my life has been laced with crisis, loss, disease and distress. And I am glad to say that I am still here, more alive, awake and energized than ever. Fortunately for me and my immune system, I have assembled a very powerful and transformative medicine bag over the years combining the ancient practices such as yoga and meditation with journal writing and expressive dance, my practical experience as an occupational therapist and the unconditional love of family and friends! Ta-Da! Shift happens. We can change! Life goes on! Like the turtle, we are already home. We just need to open the door, walk in and sit in our comfy chair!

After a series of transformative incidents and following the sudden death of my 22-year-old daughter in 2005, I made a conscious choice to change the rhythm of my life. I decided to move to what was once only a weekend getaway home on Grand Lake O' the Cherokees. Some friends advised against such a big change right after so many life-changing events. On the life-change stress scale I was off the charts. But I knew that this was a place where I could most easily relax, away from the influence of others and be nurtured by nature. Here is where the turtles began telling me their story of resilience, patience and adaptability, and calling me to tell mine. Much of my inspiration came to me as I floated in the middle of the cove on windless, warm days. Our cove is full of turtles, and the more I watched and read about them, the more I let their teachings guide me and heal me.

8

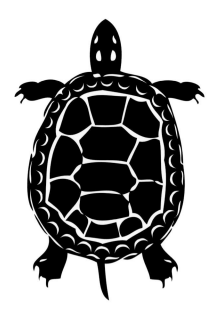

To Native Americans the turtle represents the nurturing and resilient womb of the Great Mother (God, Goddess, Universal Love), from which we all come and to which we all return (home), in life and in death. Through their example, turtles offer us simple everyday wisdom for living well:

~ Slow down

~ Be patient

~ Adapt to change

~ Be willing to stick your neck out

~ Know that you are always at home within your self

CHAPTER 1

S T A R T   W H E R E   Y O U   A R E

~ Love Your Self Enough ~

*"If a living system is suffering from ill health,
the remedy is to connect it with more of itself."*

FRANCISCO VERELA

While the idea for this book emerged several years ago, its manifestation came only after I had the opportunity to "walk my talk." I had lessons to learn and feelings and experience to integrate. I had to love myself enough to risk becoming self-employed and to walk the road less traveled in the healthcare community. I had to love myself enough to listen to my heart's desire and to create a business that would teach me as much or more than I taught others. I had to be willing to integrate my own teachings into my own life! We do teach that which we most need to learn! And so with SELF I began, and I invite you to do the same.

If you are still reading this you may be responding to a call to make changes in your lifestyle and your state of health. This may be prompted by a feeling of exhaustion, disgust, or simply a lack of comfort with your life as it is today. Or perhaps you had a recent wakeup call, an illness or a diagnosis of a disease (dis-ease), the dissolution of a relationship, the death of someone close to you or the loss of a job. In any case, you are hearing *your* call to *you*! "Hey! Pay attention to your SELF!" If you are like most of us, your tendency is to give most all of your energy away to others…your kids, your spouse, your employer, your friends and your family. Now you are being asked to stop giving all of your energy away and give some back to your self! Are you listening? If so, the news is good, because both you and those whom you love stand to benefit!

If you are really honest with yourself, your comfy chair may not be so comfortable after all. Maybe you can't remember the last time you sat there, with your SELF. You and your chair may feel pretty worn out, lumpy, saggy or just unfamiliar. You are tired, and may not feel like you have any energy to give to yourself at all! But you are here now. Your journey begins now. Now is the only *real time* we have, and every moment is like a seed, full of the potential of our fullest being.

Like the turtle, while it sometimes feels more comfortable and safe to hide in our shell we must take a little risk now and then and stick our necks out to see what is waiting around the corner. The turtle's guidance is simple and will serve as our model on this journey to everyday self-health. The first step for all of us embarking on a new path toward positive lifestyle change is to first stick our necks out. We must be willing to step out of our comfort zone, survey our options and move towards change. The good news is, like the turtle, our home is never far away! Our home is always with us. It is our inner sanctuary, our place of safety, stillness and peaceful centeredness. It is the place within. Do you remember that place? If not, I hope some of the tools presented here will help you get reacquainted with your SELF.

The *Art of Self-Health* is an integrative model for living meaningfully and living well. This model was birthed from my own burn-out in corporate healthcare and the need to create my personal medicine bag for regrouping and healing. It blends ancient energy wisdom with modern philosophy and psychology, and offers approaches for "coming home" by changing behaviors and lifestyle practices. The *Art of Self-Health* provides a model for addressing the well-being of your whole self. The practices presented here affect those parts of your self that you can see, feel, hear and touch (physical, emotional, occupational, relational, self-expressional, mental and spiritual) as well as your energy body, which is sometimes less noticeable. The steps you take toward self-health affects your energy level *and* the seven primary energy centers of the body, also known as the chakras.

The *Art of Self-Health* IS an art. It is YOUR unique process, and allows you to start where you are. It allows you to begin creating and making positive changes now that support your entire being—body, mind and spirit.

Take a moment to take stock of your current lifestyle, your comfort with your self and the love you have for your self.

♥ *Do you love your self enough* to have a sense of reverence for your physical body, honoring it through conscious daily care, nutrition, rest, relaxation and movement? (Physical Self-Health and Base Chakra)

♥ *Do you love your self enough* to consciously seek emotional freedom and pleasure through honest and authentic emotional expression? (Emotional Self-Health and Sacral Chakra)

♥ *Do you love your self enough* to acknowledge and share your unique gifts, skills and talents in your work or choice of leisure activities? (Occupational Self-Health and Solar Plexus Chakra)

♥ *Do you love your self enough* to be compassionate with yourself and to spend time and energy on YOU first in order to better nurture your relationships with family, friends and community? (Relational Self-Health and Heart Chakra)

♥ *Do you love your self enough* to listen lovingly to yourself, to express yourself creatively and to ask for what you want and need? (Self-Expressional Self-Health and Throat Chakra)

♥ *Do you love your self enough* to consciously observe and understand your thoughts and beliefs and the relationship between your thoughts and your experience? (Mental Self-Health and Third Eye Chakra)

♥ *Do you love your self enough* to quietly connect with your soul, your essence and your inner being while allowing it to guide your life with purpose and meaning? (Spiritual Self-Health and Crown Chakra)

The first step towards loving your self enough is paying attention and listening to the signals from your body/mind—tension, headaches, irritability, low energy, frequent illness, difficulty concentrating, etc. If any of these seem familiar, embrace that awareness without judgment or criticism. It is important to ***accept*** where you are now, since all change starts with self-acceptance. Cultivate awareness of your unique response to change, challenge, crisis and the demands of your life. The *Art of Self-Health* starts where you are NOW and stays where you are now, which is always changing. Love yourself enough to be patient during the inevitable setbacks! And most importantly, be willing to continue sticking out your neck to discover more of you.

13

CHAPTER 2

ANCIENT SECRETS OF A MOSAIC TURTLE

~ The Creative Process of Health ~

Soon after my daughter's sudden death I realized that there is no prescription for moving through the grieving process. I knew that I must honor my need for time to process the loss. While the world seemed to be tugging at me to live on, I felt something else. Nobody was going to tell me how to grieve. I was going to do this on my terms this time! I realized that I had let go of another child of mine 33 years earlier. When I was 17, I gave birth out of wedlock to a beautiful boy, yet I was expected to let go of him quickly. And I did. Because I felt it was the right thing to do, I gave him up for adoption and returned to high school life and cheerleading as though nothing had happened. I couldn't acknowledge or talk about it. And I definitely could not express my feelings of grief and loss. Now I was being presented with an opportunity to create my own grieving experience, to let go of a child on my own terms with consideration of my SELF. I had the opportunity to create my own path to healing. How could I know the lessons that this loss and others would teach me over the next few years?

"*Art*" implies a creative component. The ***Art** of Self-Health* supports a re-creation of self, and an opportunity to individually design your self-health by applying your personal preferences. You will be introduced to a variety of self-health tools throughout this book and it is up to you to decide which of these, or others, will best serve your personal picture of well-being. For example, a house is a basic structure with rooms, shapes, lighting and space to meet basic safety and personal aesthetic preferences. This same house may become the HOME to several different families, each designing it to meet their unique needs and comfort. While discovering and defining your self-health, I invite you to explore how your personal desires and preferences can best serve your well-being, while honoring the basic structure of wholeness, balance and self-nurturance.

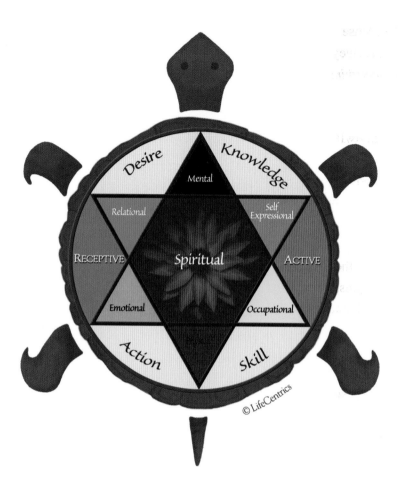

Text within the illustration: Desire, Knowledge, Mental, Relational, Self Expressional, RECEPTIVE, Spiritual, ACTIVE, Emotional, Occupational, Action, Skill, Physical, © LifeCentrics

15

Illustration A
The Art of Self-Health
A Model for Integrative Wellness

To be alive means to be productive, to use one's powers not for any purpose transcending man, but for oneself, to make sense of one's existence, to be human. As long as anyone believes that his ideal and purpose is outside himself, that it is above the clouds, in the past or in the future, he will go outside himself and seek fulfillment where it cannot be found. He will look for solutions and answers at every point except the one where they can be found…in himself.

ERICH FROMM

The Ancient Wise Turtle

Since they have inhabited the earth for millions of years, turtles have certainly been doing *something* right! Turtles exhibit many of the attributes that support self-health and longevity such as:

- the ability to adapt and change by following **desire**, obtaining **knowledge**, learning new **skills** and putting these skills into **action**.
- knowing how to balance **receptive**ness and inner focus with **active** living and outer focus.
- maintaining the strength and sturdiness of their **physical** being.
- being able to navigate changing environments and relationships like the human flow of **emotion**.
- expressing a quiet, steady confidence in their innate power, resilience and **occupation** in their earth dwelling.
- practicing the communal connection that supports **relational** well-being.
- being able to sense and respond to sound and vibration supporting their **self-expressional** being.
- practicing moving slowly, perceiving moment to moment supporting their **mental** well-being.
- simply being the **spiritual** symbol of uniting heaven and earth as represented by their shell and square underside.

Turtles are often observed congregating in communal gatherings while resting and basking in the sunlight, overlapping and stacking on top of one another. They may move through the world slowly and patiently, adapting easily to different environments and moving effortlessly from water to land. Wisely, a turtle knows he can't accomplish anything without sticking his neck out and exercising patience in the process! (Watch a turtle make its way across a road). As with any change we make in life, we need support, patience and we need to take some risk!

Just as the turtle's shell has thirteen segments, the *Art of Self-Health* model (Illustration A) has thirteen segments, (*desire, knowledge, skill, action, active, receptive, physical, emotional, occupational, relational, self-expressional, mental and spiritual.*) Native Americans taught that the thirteen segments on the shell of the turtle represent *natural time* and the annual cycle of either thirteen new moons or full moons. So with the turtle as our guide, we will approach self-health from the perspective of returning to our *natural* state of balance while honoring our individual sense of timing and engagement.

16

This model for the *Art of Self-Health* (Illustration B) is full of symbolism. Let's begin with the circle. The circle containing the thirteen segments represents our inherent wholeness. A circle has no beginning and no end. It symbolizes life as a continuous, ongoing process, always returning to the beginning—our SELF. The circle represents the womb of the Great Mother, new beginnings, safety and limitless possibility. It means that any change or action on our part in *any* dimension of our being can potentially touch, and transform the bigger circle and the whole of the universe. The circle represents community and connectedness. Our circle of friends and family provides the container of support, love and belonging that nurtures our wholeness and our sense of completeness within our selves.

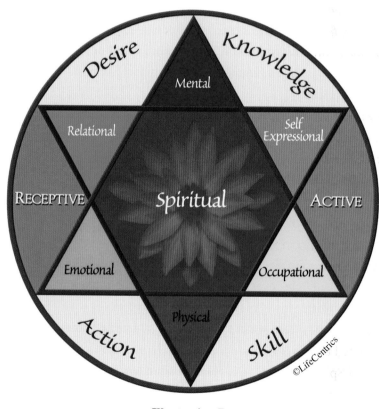

Illustration B

17

The circle also represents the wheel of positive change. Lifestyle changes are driven by our **desire**, the acquisition of **knowledge** and the integration of new **skills** and **action** in daily life. Change is also supported by times of being overtly **active** and times of inner focus and being more **receptive**. As you change, your relationship with your world may change. Relationships with your spouse, your children, your friends and perhaps even your employer may shift. Our experiences and discoveries change our perceptions, our feelings and our actions. Any simple or positive shift which allows you to find more joy and energy every day will not only transform you, but will positively influence your family, your co-workers, your friends, and in some small but significant way, the world.

For several years I chose (with my husband at the time) to be the primary bread winner for the family while our two children were in grade school and middle school. It was a non-traditional lifestyle for our social circle, and the PTA women certainly loved the involvement of the stay-at-home dad! I was making more money than I ever thought possible using my skills mostly as a manager, with little application of my hands-on clinical skills as an occupational therapist. Our family enjoyed the lucrative income and the freedom it afforded us, but because of the toll the job was taking on my health, marriage, family and creativity, I needed to make a change. I desired to pursue something in the field of holistic health, an area of healthcare I had studied on my own for some time. Needless to say, the change that I made had profound effects on the whole family. Our lifestyle and our priorities soon shifted, but it was wonderful to later watch my children pursue interests in areas for which they had a passion instead of what would bring in the biggest paycheck! I would like to believe that the choices I made positively influenced those in my circle. This I know—I am certainly happier and healthier, and that is definitely good for those around me.

Have no doubt that during your own journey toward everyday self-health you may affect and change more than yourself. And that is potentially a very good thing! For as you grow into more pleasure, power and purpose there is more to give and more for others to receive. We *all* feel better. Your positive change can influence the circle of the whole.

Next, let's look at the symbolism of the triangles. The triangle with the apex at the top (pointed upward) represents the age-old trinity (Father, Son and Holy Spirit, Mind, Body and Spirit, or the Triple Goddess—maiden, mother and crone.) It is also the symbol of masculine or active energy, energy that is grounded and stable on the earth yet focused and moving outward toward heaven. The triangle with the apex at the bottom (pointed downward) represents feminine or receptive energy. This is the chalice, the cup, the vessel that is open to receiving and holding. Feminine energy is flowing and non-linear. We need both feminine and masculine energy for balance. The equilateral triangle in itself is a symbol of balance, all sides equal, all aspects of our being equally important.

Within the circle on the back of the turtle, the two intersecting triangles create the **six-pointed star**, housing the seven dimensions of well-being. In the center of the star is a solid, spacious hexagram connecting our **spiritual** dimension to the points radiating outward (**physical, emotional, occupational, relational, self-expressional and mental**). The center hexagram and the lotus flower within is a symbol of our comfy chair, our place of centeredness. Within this center is our most quiet and still point of peacefulness, and our point of infinite possibility. Each facet of outward manifestation is in itself a trinity, a balanced triangle of body, mind and spirit, connected to and fueled by our center of spiritual essence. We are already whole and balanced. But like a rainbow, it takes light to reveal and illuminate the full spectrum of rich color within. Think of giving attention to your self and your state of well-being as standing fully in the light so your brightest colors can shine.

CHAPTER 3

B A L A N C E
~ Supporting Change through Equilibrium ~

Whatever you receive, wherever it comes from,
cherish the desire to give it back in full measure.

SWAMI CHIDVILASANANDA

*A few years ago I was living a dream. After leaving corporate healthcare, I followed my heart's desire, took a risk and borrowed some money to start my own business. I created and opened a center that offered movement classes and workshops that supported mind, body and spirit. I was teaching what I know and love, dancing every day while providing a place for individuals and groups to be supported, healthy and joyful. Wow! Such a deal! However, after five years, I realized that I was tired. Even though I was loving my work and teaching what I was passionate about, I was **doing** too much and not **receiving** enough emotionally, financially, mentally and spiritually. My mistake was thinking I was immune to burn-out because I was **doing** work I loved. Yet the reality was that I was giving, giving, giving and leaving little or no time for my own receiving and learning. My cup was emptying faster than it was filling up. I had lost balance, even while doing what I loved every day.*

Health is enhanced when we achieve and maintain a state of equilibrium and balance. As seen in the circle (Illustration B), the *Art of Self-Health* includes the **Receptive** left side of the circle and the **Active** right side of the circle. In Chinese medicine, these receptive and active aspects of our being are referred to as the **Yin** and **Yang**. Each is balanced by, surrounds and contains the other.

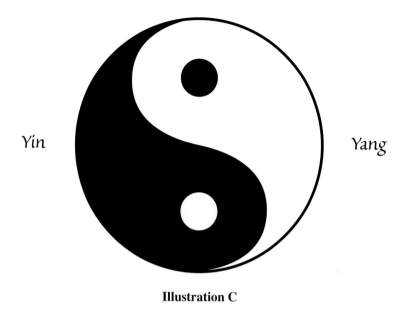

Yin

Yang

Illustration C

As **Masculine** energy is active, giving and outward focused, Chinese medicine refers to this as **Yang** energy. **Yang** or **Active** energy is controlled by the left hemisphere of the brain and controls the right side of the body. The active component is on the right side of the turtle model. In humans, the left side of the brain controls the right side of the body. The left side of the brain is associated with linear, organized thinking, like balancing a checkbook or formulating a specific plan for a improving your health.

The polar opposite of Yang energy is **Yin** energy, or the **Feminine** aspect of self. **Yin** or **Receptive** energy is controlled by the right side of the brain, which controls the left side of the body. The receptive component is on the left side of the model. The right hemisphere of the brain influences our spatial and creative thinking, like arranging flowers in a vase, painting a picture or listening to and following inspiration for a new class to take.

The natural state of our being is balance. As infants we enter this world with an inner knowing and tendency to seek balance, an innate rhythm of **activity** and **receptivity**. As babies, we generally demand and receive enough nourishment to support our energy expenditure, mental activity and physical growth. Yin and Yang are reflected in the following characteristics.

Yin Energy	Yang Energy
Still	Moving
Dark	Light
Receptive	Active
Moon	Sun
Inner	Outer
Non-linear	Linear
Able to Let Go	Controlling
Creative	Directive

In today's times our society and culture often demand an over-expression of Yang energy. Value is placed on achievement, active socialization, multi-tasking, immediate gratification and doing more and more. These societal expectations require an almost constant expenditure of energy into the world. Because the majority of the American work force is in the service industry, we are continually asked to give, give and give of our skills, knowledge and hearts in the workplace, receiving little more than a paycheck in return.

Our nervous systems have become accustomed to and oftentimes addicted to the "on" mode of operation. When our bodies demand rest and sleep, we have difficulty quieting our minds and allowing that nurturance. Resting and relaxing consciously—taking a nap or just sitting and doing nothing—is often perceived as lazy and unproductive, even though it helps return our energy to a state of balance.

Too Much of a Good Thing…When Balance Breaks

~ TURTLE WISDOM ~

When a turtle gets too hot, it moves into the water and maybe deep into the cool mud below. It chooses an environment that soothes, rejuvenates and provides a sense of buoyancy and support.

No matter what you are doing in life, if you do *too much, too fast*, for *too long* you will experience burnout. Our internal rhythms are seductively influenced by the perceived mandates of the outside world and our perceived need to do more and have more. Sadly, we begin to think that the daily headaches, sleepless nights and chronic irritability are normal. And as the pharmaceutical industry is all too ready to remind us, there is always a pill that will help! Everyday living can become rote and mechanical. The juices of creativity, passion, deep love and laughter can cease to flow, leaving us feeling parched and empty. We find ourselves simply going through the motions while meeting the ever-increasing demands of boss, customers, family and friends. We are running on adrenaline-fueled energy and auto-pilot.

The *Art of Self Health* asks us to design more space in our lives for **yin** energy. It asks us to seek and create a balance of doing and not doing, giving and receiving, focusing on our inner landscape as much as we focus on the outer world. For many of us this requires a major shift in our values and core beliefs. It also may require giving up or letting go of the illusion that we can control anyone or anything outside of ourselves.

It is important to recognize the real possibility of physical, mental, emotional and spiritual depletion that occurs from perpetual motion and rigorous activity—*doing*. We must also realize that we can best serve, love and care for those in our world from a place of fullness. We must fill our own cup first, only then will we have enough to share with others. Filling our own cup, however, requires valuing our selves, taking time for self-nurturing and allowing others to give to us. This may require us to consciously give up control, sit in the stillness and be open to receiving the love and support that is around us but may have gone unnoticed in all of our busyness! Then we can create the beautiful cycle of giving and receiving, active and inactive, holding and letting go—BALANCE.

Many research studies have emerged lately touting the health benefits of vitamin D. Our bodies naturally manufacture vitamin D as a result of exposure to sunlight. Scientists say it is good to receive unprotected sun rays on our skin for up to ten minutes a day. I find it interesting that we are being encouraged to RECEIVE (yin) the SUN (yang) energy in support of our health. Simply *receive*.

As you move toward creating positive change in each of the seven dimensions of well-being, which are, physical, emotional, occupational, relational, self-expressional mental and spiritual, you are encouraged to include in *your* design for self-health a balance of energy out and energy in. You and your physical vessel (your body) are like a battery. There is a lot more running time on a fully charged battery, but the battery must be willing to take in the energy as well as give it away.

23

Awareness Activity

Take a moment to list examples of your typical "Yang" life activities. In what ways are you "out there" planning, giving and doing everyday?

Next, list examples of your typical "Yin" life activities. In what ways do you regularly pause and receive nurturance and inspiration?

24

Which is the longer list?

What can you and are you willing to change about the imbalance?

CHAPTER 4

CHANGE IS NATURAL

~ Water, Earth, Fire and Air ~

Change means movement.

Movement means friction.

SAUL ALINSKY

Observe and sense your natural surroundings. Change is an integral part of the natural world. The art of creating self-health is a dynamic process fueled by four stages of positive behavioral change: *desire, knowledge, skill and action*. Change is a component of any transformation. In the natural world, change is both fueled and tamed by the elements *water, earth, fire and air*. All four stages and all four natural elements are essential to the art of recreating ourselves and changing the state of our self-health.

Stage of Change	Nature's Element	Influence on Personal Self-Health
DESIRE	WATER	MOVEMENT
KNOWLEDGE	EARTH	SUBSTANCE
SKILL	FIRE	TRANSFORMATION
ACTION	AIR	EXPANSION/INSPIRATION

Awareness and the will to consciously create change is the foundation for self-health. To create any change in our lives, it's important to possess, activate and integrate each of these key stages and elements. They are the foundation and the structure for reclaiming balance and equilibrium in our lives.

While change is a fundamental element of personal growth and expansion, many of us resist and avoid it. Proactively creating change in our lives takes courage, faith, adaptability and commitment. Many people do not believe they have the power to create positive change. Typically, they allow outside circumstances, situations or people to instigate change for them. *"I got fired from my job"* or *"The stock market is not letting me retire on time."* They view change as out of their control. *"This situation happened to me, so I had to make a change."*

~ TURTLE WISDOM ~

The turtle roams the shoreline searching for food and sustenance. When it realizes that none is to be found there, it simply **changes** *its search to the water, slipping gracefully and patiently into the cool, fluid depths that will feed it.*

The natural world teaches us a lot about rhythms of transformation for the purpose of maintaining balance. The key elements of the natural world, (*earth, water, fire and air*) are interrelated and represent different characteristics of change. The key is balance, and integrating all elements in balance can keep us grounded, passionate, sensitive and light-hearted!

Creating self-health may require changing core beliefs and values, changing habits, changing attitudes, changing relationships, changing activities and perhaps even changing jobs or careers. The journey of change is not for the faint of heart. In order for change to have both meaning and a profound life benefit, it must be illuminated with the heart's *desire*. The heart's desire is the beacon illuminating the path of the seeker. Change requires us to move from a place that feels secure, safe and familiar (earth element), into a place that is fluid and sometimes deep and ever changing (water element). *The turtle does this easily and effortlessly!* How will we know that greater comfort is only a step away unless we take that first step into the unknown? How will we know that we cannot create a more vibrant self unless we *stick our necks out* and take the risk of trying?

Stages of Lifestyle Change

The four stages of lifestyle change are:
- **Desire (Water Element)** - "I want to feel good."
- **Knowledge (Earth Element)** - "I am willing to learn and acquire the information I need to manifest my desire."
- **Skill (Fire Element)** - "I am willing to try something new, dedicate time and practice, and learn from my mistakes."

- **Action (Air Element)** - "I am willing to put positive changes into action demonstrating care for my self, family, community, workplace and the world."

NATURE'S ELEMENTAL BALANCE

Element	Change Characteristic	Balancing Remedy
Water	Too much water energy can result in unclear emotional and physical boundaries, constant change, diluted and unclear feelings.	**Fire:** *Expressing personal strength and power* can vaporize excessive water energy and can dilute overwhelming emotions **Earth:** *Connecting with the body* can use sensation to impose a safe structure, boundaries, grounding and focus on the now **Air:** *Deep breathing* can lighten the intensity of emotions
Earth	Too much earth energy results in feeling stuck, immobile, heavy, boxed in, and too comfortable, making change difficult.	**Air:** *Deep breathing and laughter* moves lightness into the body **Fire:** Ignite change by *trying something new* which can break inertia and transform old habits and patterns **Water:** *Emote and express your feelings* which can provide a sense of cleansing and washing away of the old structures and staleness
Fire	Too much fire energy can lead to excessive movement and activity, burnout and lack of focus. Too little fire energy can lead to lethargy, stagnation, lack of passionate pursuits.	**Water:** Focus on *flowing, sensing, observing, and enjoying the moment* which can provide a sense of soothing coolness **Earth:** Indulge in *physical sensation and pleasure such as massage or sex* which can provide grounding and ignite passion **Air:** *Deep breathing and inspiration* can be enlivening and transformative to a smoldering fire
Air	Too much air energy results in excessive thinking and talking. Feeling flighty, light-headed, and indecisive can result in limited focus, confusion and anxiety, "paralysis by analysis."	**Earth:** Ground yourself through *sensing, experiencing and listening to the physical body* **Fire:** Warm to expanded possibilities by *moving into and focusing on something you are passionate about* **Water:** *Focus on your feelings and the bodily sensation of emotions* which can provide density and form

28

Let's consider each one of these stages in greater depth.

Desire

*Your desire is your prayer. Picture the fulfillment of your desire now
and feel its reality and you will experience the joy of the
answered prayer.*

DR. JOSEPH MURPHY

Inherent in the core of our being is the *desire* for pleasure. Who doesn't want to feel good? Through desire we create movement and change in our lives. The word *emotion* (*E*-motion) means giving *energy* (E) to *movement* (motion), or *moving energy*. Water is the element of emotion. The desire for pleasure is what initially breaks through stagnation and inertia (earth). Through movement, we create change. Consciously creating change that supports our well-being begins with giving attention to the *desire* to change. In terms of our physical health, we may desire to have more energy, perhaps fueled by a pleasant memory of feeling vital, energetic and strong a few years or a few short months ago. Our own bodily and cell memories can influence our desire in both positive and negative ways. For example, tap into a memory of a time when you felt loved, energetic, powerful, beautiful, intelligent, etc. Then ask your cells to energetically recapture and carry forward that memory to the present. More than likely, just thinking about that time of your life you will begin feeling good, and feeling good will fuel the desire to keep feeling good! On the other hand, if when you felt peaceful, calm and quiet someone close to you called you *lazy*, your cells carry that memory of negative judgment. It may then be difficult to arouse the desire to practice relaxation again, for fear of being called lazy.

When choosing to consciously create positive change in our personal system of *self-health*, sometimes the most difficult step is awakening our desire. It certainly takes less energy, and little or no movement (emotion) to simply settle for the status quo. Consciously awakening our desire for change involves being willing to risk the unfamiliar, and to consciously reprogram our attunement to what we desire. Conscious desire for change not only fuels positive change for ourselves, but through our change, we influence our world (family, friends or coworkers) in positive ways. It's simply the **ripple effect**, the water energy of desire!

29

Choosing from Love or Fear

Our deepest fear is not that we are inadequate.
Our deepest fear is that we are powerful beyond measure.
It is our light, not our darkness that most frightens us.
And as we let our own light shine, we unconsciously give other people
permission to do the same. As we are liberated from our fear,
our presence automatically liberates others.

Excerpts from NELSON MANDELA, 1994 Inaugural Speech

Unfortunately, fear is what initiates the desire and process of change in many of us. If change is fueled primarily by *fear*, it begins from a place of constriction and limitation. We often begin to make changes with fear based beliefs such as "If I don't quit smoking, I will get lung cancer," or "If I quit this job I hate I won't be able to find another job and I will go broke," or "If I don't exercise I will develop heart disease." But it is our desires that come from love—love for your SELF and your self-health that provides the most pervasive, long-lasting catalyst for positive change. When I experience or think of fear, I see and feel darkness and cold. When I experience or think of love, I see and feel warmth and light. The "freeze" created by fear is thawed by love. ***Where there is love, there is no room for fear***. If you begin with loving your self and allow that to initiate and infiltrate your every desire, you will create an open space for healing and for long-lasting well-being. The previous statements change to "I want healthy lungs and freedom from addiction," or "I want to enjoy my job and the work I do everyday," and "I want to enjoy a strong heart and increased energy from exercising everyday."

*I had a small vacation home on a lake in northeastern Oklahoma for 10 years. When I spent time there it became more and more difficult for me to return to the city and the long work weeks. My deepest desire was to wake up to the natural, peaceful beauty of the lake every day while making a living doing what I loved and knew how to do. I desired a steady stream of income while enjoying freedom and flexibility! That was the seed of desire that fueled my move to the lake full time in 2006. It was the desire to move **toward** something I loved and that filled my soul. When that desire bubbled up inside me, I didn't have all the details of "how" figured out yet, but I somehow knew that if I took the first step, the details would be revealed. While it took a couple of years to take that step, I stayed committed to the call of a slower and more mindful rhythm of living. I knew that the call was for loving my self more deeply. After all, what's the worst thing that*

30

could happen? I could always move back to the city. So, here I am, living the life of my desire. Every day I wake up and breathe in the natural beauty of this place, and I am grateful to the depths of my soul.

Getting in touch with desire through love sometimes requires examining and reprogramming our basic beliefs. Thinking "I don't deserve," "I have no power," "I am not worthy," or "What I want is not important" can derail any movement toward positive change. These core beliefs must first be acknowledged, and then consciously shifted to allow *self love* to be the true seed for our desire. (See **Appendix L**, page 170) Our path to balanced living, to self-health, begins with creating a statement of desire that supports self-health from self-love. Are you ready to let the flow of change begin? Start where you are now, with writing a personal desire statement.

EXAMPLE:
Desire statement: "I desire the ability to relax and let go of worry"

Love energy: "I love the feeling of inner peace and the positive effect relaxation has on my relationships and work."

31

┌─────────────── PERSONAL APPLICATION ───────────────┐

Connect with your Desire: Take a moment to close your eyes and sit quietly for a moment while observing your breath. Silently ask yourself, "What is one thing that I desire that would help me feel better?"

Infuse the desire with love: Now reflect for a moment on how this desire is an expression of love for your self.

└──┘

Knowledge

It is not because things are difficult that we do not dare;
it is because we do not dare that they are difficult.

SENECA

The next stage of positive behavioral change and creating your *Art of Self-Health* is *knowledge*. Acquiring the knowledge we need is the first step in transforming our desire into positive change. Knowledge is the earth element from which we create change. It brings focus and structure to the water energy and movement of desire. Acquiring knowledge can be the process of allowing ourselves to *remember*. We all possess the knowledge of past experience. Many of us can remember a time of balance, optimum health and joy. Our knowing has simply been masked by long episodes of operating on auto pilot, muddling through the daily chaos, being unaware and in a state of stagnation and inertia. We are just like a turtle stuck in the mud!

Acquiring knowledge requires activating and nurturing of the mind. The emotional energy of desire must meld with the place where we assemble information, store memory and imagine possibilities. We must open our minds to visualizing, remembering and learning. And while seeking the information we need, we must also be willing to still our minds long enough to be self-observant and filter the tendency towards "information overload."

Our resources for knowledge are vast, and can sometimes seem overwhelming. We have access to a world-wide web of information via the internet on every subject imaginable. When seeking the knowledge to support our desire for positive change, we must be discerning and avoid the tendency to move into a place of "paralysis by analysis." Too much information can be paralyzing, and can feel like being loaded down with a ton of rocks (earth). *"I don't know where to start!"* Once again, the heart can be our guide in choosing the particular media, teacher, philosophy, resource and information we need to support changes toward self-health.

The saying "when the student is ready, the teacher will appear" holds very true for this aspect of change. If your desire is true to your heart and guided by self-love, you will attract the precise information you need, in the form best suited for your learning. Here is a personal example:

In 1998 I was a high-level manager in a corporate rehabilitation and healthcare system and it was taking a toll on my health and my family. Although I was making great money, I am a "people person" who found herself managing bottom-line *financial performance, traveling a lot, losing sleep and feeling tired, anxious and unfulfilled. Other than the occasional walk or exercise class I was far out of touch with caring for my whole self, something I believed we should all do more. My core beliefs and outward practices were clearly incongruent. I had literally quit "dancing," finding little or no joy in my movement through life. I thought "surely people's health and well-being can be more proactively influenced, and I want to have something to do with that!" As yet another corporate buyout and restructuring occurred (the fourth in four years), I saw an opportunity to make the leap out of the corporate world. I stepped into the unknown with a short severance package and the desire to practice wellness and health promotion from a holistic perspective. I had this heartfelt desire, yet I wasn't clear what I would do or how I would do it, a huge part of the **knowledge** piece!*

One morning I was sitting at the kitchen table and turned to my favorite section of the newspaper. On the front page was a picture of a woman doing a karate kick of sorts with a joyous facial expression. This was a syndicated article featuring an exercise form called The Nia Technique®, or Nia (pronounced nee-ah). As I read further about its "mind, body, spirit, emotion" focus and its combination of the dance arts, martial arts and healing arts, I felt tears welling in my eyes and goose bumps all over my body! I thought "Wow! This is holistic fitness and the perfect way to combine my love of dance, my occupational therapy background and helping others become healthy."

It took some searching (calling the studio in Philadelphia where the picture was taken and eventually calling the Nia headquarters in Portland) to discover there wasn't anyone close to me in Kansas City who taught this technique. Taking a live class was next to impossible, so I ordered a video. I fell in love with the technique and signed up for a week long intensive training without having taken a real class. My source of knowledge serendipitously appeared and my life was soon transformed. During that week of intensive training I cried a lot, moving emotions and energy that had been stuck for years. I also felt like a part of me had "come home."

"*When the student is ready, the teacher will appear.*" Sometimes finding the information you need takes searching, and sometimes it falls in your lap, simply because you have experienced the desire.

Possible knowledge sources to support "*I desire the ability to relax and let go of worry*" would include:
- Internet search on the benefits of meditation and relaxation.
- Books, tapes, CDs on relaxation.
- Classes and training in relaxation with biofeedback.
- Teacher, trainer or life coach for clarifying values and time

management for relaxation.

- Fun loving friends who teach through playing, relaxing and experiencing.

Sometimes finding the knowledge is the easy part and becoming the open-minded student is what requires the commitment and energy. Simply start where you are and watch as your field of information and knowledge expands one small step at a time.

> ━━ PERSONAL APPLICATION ━━
>
> **Knowledge Sources:** Take a moment to reflect on the resources at your disposal for gaining the knowledge to support your desire. Is there someone in your circle of support who you can question or seek guidance from? Make a list of your possible resources. *Maybe working through this book is your first step!*

Skill

When people make changes in their lives in a certain area,
they may start by changing the way they talk about that subject,
how they act about it, their attitude toward it,
or an underlying decision concerning it.

JANE ILLSLEY CLARK

Skill requires integration of mind, body and emotion. Developing skill is the next step in creating positive change in our self-health. Skill development requires the transformative energy of the element of fire. When you combine desire and knowledge, or water and earth, you can create a form out of the resulting mud or clay. A ceramic pot, formed from clay (earth and water) only becomes a substantial, strong container after it is "fired" in a kiln. Skill is the integration of our desire and our knowledge, bringing desire and knowledge into physical manifestation. This is the step where we infuse our cells and molecules with our knowing.

Skill development is our practice ground. It is the place where we can actually begin the transformation and *feel* the change that we desire. This *feeling* now becomes our teacher. We begin to know more through the art of doing, and doing *consciously*. Practicing a new activity asks that we periodically move into the role of *observer* and the role of observer demands that we look at ourselves objectively. We may need to ask "What is working? What is not working? What is causing me to feel good? What is causing me to feel tense or constricted?" What we observe may require us to shift our application of the knowledge we have gathered.

Skill development is the stage of change that requires the greatest commitment of time and energy. Studies show that it takes from 21-66 days for new behaviors to become habits and the transformation to take hold. Skill development requires constant practice, self observation, knowledge application, adjustment and allowing integration. We must repeatedly practice the skill and repeatedly feel good while doing it before we are ready to move out into the world with the new behavior. Change has manifested! Transformation has occurred!

*In November1999 during my initial training in The Nia Technique®, I remember feeling like I had "come home" to myself. While the skill of Nia was brand new, the cells in my body were infused all week with **feelings** of joy, relief, belonging and expectation. The skill integration had begun, and it felt good and easy because I was learning a skill that felt natural and life-supporting!*

35

Possible steps in skill development for: "I desire the ability to relax and let go of worry."
* Learn deep belly breathing. See The Conscious Breath, page 54.
* Commit to disengaging your cell phone and computer at home in the evenings.
* Set aside 10 minutes each evening for alone time.
* During alone time listen to a short guided meditation tape.
* Take time after the tape to observe how you feel. Record feelings in a journal.
* Try different tapes and observe differences in how you feel.
* Practice belly breathing at morning, noon and afternoon work breaks.
* Expand quiet relaxation time to 20 minutes or 10 minutes in the morning and 10 minutes in the evening.
* Practice doing nothing (sitting outside in nature, sitting and listening to music) with someone whom you love or whose company you enjoy.
* Notice the positive changes in your relationships, work, etc. as you practice relaxation daily.
* Every time your "observer" catches you worrying, pause and breathe deeply.

■ PERSONAL APPLICATION ■

Skill Development: Review your desire that is infused with love and the sources of knowledge you have at your disposal. Now make a list of ways that you will put into motion and practice the knowledge and information you have. Be sure to start with "practice sessions" that are absolutely doable and that you can accommodate into your life NOW.

Action

Whatever you think you can do or believe you can do, begin it.
Action has magic, grace and power in it.

JOHANN WOLFGANG VON GOETHE

Action is the art of *expanding* the life changes that support self-health and carrying those changes into everyday living. The air element associated with action fuels personal expansion and lightness in our lives. Right *action* is behavior or activity charged with the energy to support our path on the high road. Living in right *action* integrates the energy and experiences of *desire*, *knowledge* and *skill* into practical everyday application. Right action supports our truest, cleanest being and our highest purpose. This is the phase of our self-health walk that brings us into alignment with living in a meaningful way. By integrating the smallest change into right *action*, like drinking more water instead of soda or pausing to breathe deeply throughout each day, we are expanding our own self-health. We are also seeding positive planetary transformation through our personal transformation and our every breath. Right action feels like a long, slow, exhale (there's that air again) and relaxation into our truest being.

Through action, our earthly vessel (body) becomes the carrier of the self-health practices we have chosen through our desire (emotion), our knowledge (mind) and our skill development (body, mind, emotion integration) for purpose and meaning (spirit). As we integrate our self-health changes, it continues to be important to step into the observer role and ask ourselves, "How is this action in alignment with my core beliefs and values and how does it serve my highest good?"

While focus and discipline are necessary components of any behavior or activity change, so are light-heartedness and joy. We will know that our action is "right" by noticing how we feel while incorporating and *being* this behavior or activity change in everyday life. Our action may be a daily or weekly ritual and eventually we may actually feel *pulled* into the action because it just won't feel right if we don't do it! It may feel as natural as brushing your teeth or kissing your kids goodnight. Right action embodies a feeling of effortlessness, lightness and ease. Right action manifests as a feeling of connectedness to our self, others and the universe as a whole.

I returned from my training in The Nia Technique® to a community ready for its teachings. From day one, I felt completely supported by the universe as I aligned with my "right action." The first Nia classes in Kansas City were well attended from day one and over the next few years a supportive community of students and friends evolved. The Saturday morning classes in particular held a more spiritual focus and I felt something was missing when I didn't teach or participate in those. I found myself doing something I loved, positively influencing the health and well-being of others and belonging to a community of people full of love and support for one another. This right action of dancing and experiencing pleasure by moving my body continues to this day as I practice and infuse joyful, pleasurable movement into all of my workshops and retreats. Embodying my teachings through movement and dance is my right action.

While the word "action" implies *doing*, in the *Art of Self-Health* action may mean choosing to NOT DO. Right action may be the act of letting go of something (a belief or behavior) that does not support one's highest good. For example, drinking more water each day may require stopping the consumption of diet soda or coffee. Pausing to take deep breaths throughout the day requires letting go of busy-ness, both physically and mentally.

> ## PERSONAL APPLICATION
>
> ***Action:*** Think of a daily or weekly habit or that gives you a sense of joy, peace or fulfillment. Reflect now on how this right action developed into being an integral part of your life. How can you apply that same process, feeling or experience to creating a *new* right action to support your current self-health?

These four stages of positive behavioral change—*desire, knowledge, skill and action*—apply to any change we choose to make in our everyday life. Sometimes change will take a day, sometimes months or years. Sometimes change is suddenly forced on us, by the sudden loss of a loved one, the loss of a job or a move from a home. Sometimes change is a seductive or subtle transformation that gradually occurs as the result of increased awareness and paying attention to our lives and our choices. Every dimension of our lives is a possible canvas for change and re-creation. Our role is being willing to explore, discover and adapt. Does change create a sense of *despair* or *discovery* within you? If you choose discovery, let's begin your discovery of self-health. Remember, it is *your choices* that create your *Art of Self-Health*.

CHAPTER 5

THE HEALING POWER OF SEVEN
~ Seven Chakras and Seven Dimensions of Self-Health ~

When you really listen to yourself, you can heal yourself.

CEANNE DEROHAN

Throughout history, the number seven has been significant in various religions, mythology, anatomy, chemistry and biology. Seven virtues, seven days in week, seven vertebrae in a mammal's neck, seven chakras, the Seven Wonders of the World, etc. The *Art of Self-Health* includes a multi-colored six-pointed star containing seven distinct yet interrelated dimensions of well-being. They are ***physical, emotional, occupational, relational, self-expressional, mental and spiritual***. The colors associated with each dimension represent the seven colors in the full spectrum of light, or the rainbow, just as the seven dimensions represent the full, integrated expression of our being. Full spectrum living is balanced living. Attention to each dimension is essential in creating our unique mosaic of living, or *Art of Self-Health*. While the sum of the parts create the whole, we each must discover for ourselves, and choose for ourselves, when, how and how much attention we give to each dimension of our being. It is important to recognize that the art of our life is a balancing act, an act of continuous recreation. While we would all love to have our lives fall into perfect order and balance, it is a pretty unrealistic expectation considering the rapid change and unpredictability in our world, our relationships and our responsibilities to ourselves and others. While we may feel pretty "together" in our work or professional dimension of our life, we may be having issues with our body weight or a key relationship with a friend or spouse may be falling apart, requiring our energy and attention. Creating balance in the dimensions of our lives is a constant dance of awareness, intention and attention. Creating self-health requires conscious self-observation, setting intentions for change and giving attention to those intentions.

In the *Art of Self-Health* the seven dimensions and colors of each correlate to the seven energy centers of the body, or ***chakras***. Chakra is a Sanskrit word meaning wheel and the chakras are an ancient form of energy wisdom linked with the science and

40

practice of yoga. Yoga is a 5,000 year old practice of body alignment, breathing and meditation that is designed to connect or "yoke" the mortal self to its divine nature of pure consciousness. In relation to the body, these chakras or energy centers lie along the spinal column from the base of the spine (base chakra/physical dimension/red) to the crown of the head (crown chakra/spiritual dimension/violet). Men and women have the same chakras. Each of these energy centers is affected by both our emotions and our thoughts. They connect and influence our nerves, hormones and physical body. Based on its location along the spinal column, each chakra, or energy center, influences the vitality of the corresponding organs and body parts. For example, the first, or base chakra, correlates with the lower spine and vertebrae and influences the nerves that control the legs and feet, as well as our feelings of security and safety. So feeling stuck or issues with body weight may represent a lack of balance in the base chakra. Chakra energy can be under-active or over-active. The example above of feeling stuck or overweight may indicate too much stability and security in the base chakra.

41

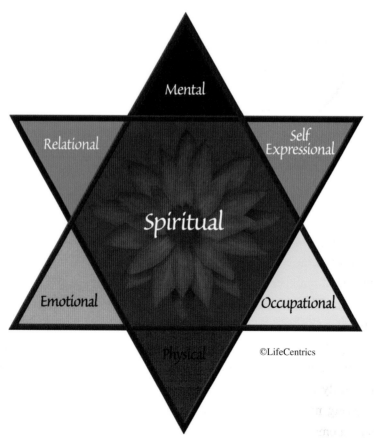

©LifeCentrics

Seven Dimensions of Well-Being

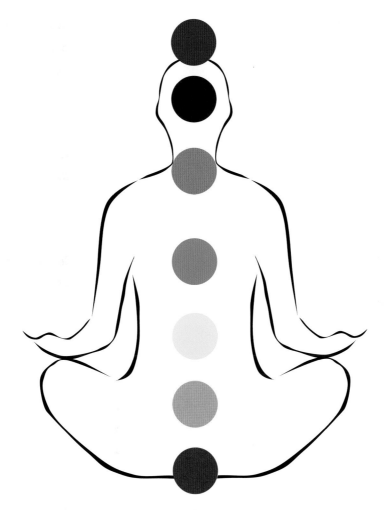

Seven Chakras

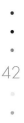

Integrating the wisdom of our energy body (chakras) with everyday practical choices can create a fulfilling, healthful and balanced life. The seven chakras and the seven dimensions of our being create a profound and powerful formula for wholeness, integrating the mind, body and spirit.

Eastern cultures have long honored the seven chakras as a system where emotional energy transforms to influence the health and vitality of the physical body. Western medicine is only beginning to appreciate the influence of energy on the body, and has yet to fully recognize the chakra system. In recent years, however, modern medicine is giving more and more credibility to the mind/body connection and the influence that our emotional and mental energy has on our physical health and longevity. For some, chakras and energy may be a difficult concept to grasp. Yet we all know and have felt the simple energetic connection between a thought (worry about finances) and a sensation in our bodies (tension headache). This is an example of the related energy of the sixth chakra (located at the center of the brow) and mental self-health.

The *Art of Self-Health* model illustrates that all of the dimensions and all of the chakras are interdependent. That is, any change or enhancement in any dimension or energy center of your body will affect the others. For example, as you make a change in expressing your self more truthfully and openly, (throat chakra/self-expressional self-health) the health of your relationships will change (heart chakra/relational self-health.) We are indeed dynamic, creative beings, capable of manifesting and radiating enormous personal power!

The locations of the seven chakras have a direct relationship to our spinal column and our nervous system. The energy of the chakras directly influence our circulatory system, our organs, our muscles and even our skin. **Appendix Q** on pages 181-182 gives examples of the corresponding body parts and how they can be affected when a chakra is out of balance.

43

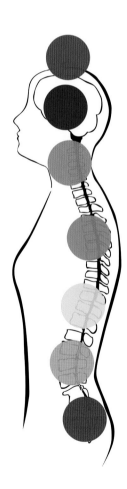

Relationship of Seven Chakras to the Vertebrae

In remembering and recreating our individual paths to self-health, we will incorporate the ancient science and wisdom of the chakra system with the practical application of everyday life changes to positively impact the seven dimensions of self-health. Through blending the ancient chakra system and modern wisdom and tools we can consciously create a meaningful transformation of our everyday energy into greater vibrancy and vitality. As the turtle model shows, the spiritual aspect of our well-being (the lotus flower in the center) touches and influences every dimension of our self-health. This dimension can be experienced as a very small, still, peaceful place within (our center), or it can be experienced as larger than life, infinite, all connecting and all expansive. Love is the center and core of every thing and SELF is where all love must begin. When you love your self, you are just as comfortable being quiet, still, alone and inward-focused as you are serving, relating and sharing love. You could say it is the he*art* of our wholeness. In the he*art* of our self-health, our healing must begin with *unconditional self-love*. The process of transformation begins with accepting and loving yourself where you are and being able to sit, if only briefly, in your comfy chair and listen honestly to your heart's desire. It takes a willingness to state even the simplest desire out loud to yourself, surrounding your desire with a feeling of love for yourself, here and now. Creating your *Art of Self-Health* will require time, energy and attention. You are encouraged to allow your blossoming into greater well-being to occur naturally and organically. *Simply put, start where you are, love your self where you are, and allow your love for your self to transform you and your world with pleasure, power and purpose!*

Self-Assessment

Take a moment now to complete the ***Art of Self-Health* Checklist** on the following page. While most responses are not clearly Yes or No, go with your first instinct in response to the statements. It may be tempting to answer yes because you have done this in the past, but be honest with yourself and answer WHERE YOU ARE NOW. Pay particular attention to those dimensions where you answer No to two or more statements. These may be areas that need your attention. *Awareness* and *balance* are the keys!

44

Art of Self-Health Checklist

Physical Self-Health and Base Chakra

• I practice some form of moderate exercise regularly.   ☐ Yes   ☐ No

• I eat a primarily natural and nutritional diet.   ☐ Yes   ☐ No

• I get 7-8 hours of sleep a night.   ☐ Yes   ☐ No

• I practice deep, abdominal breathing to relax.   ☐ Yes   ☐ No

Emotional Self-Health and Sacral Chakra

• I feel and express emotions easily.   ☐ Yes   ☐ No

• I laugh often.   ☐ Yes   ☐ No

• I am honest with myself.   ☐ Yes   ☐ No

• I allow myself to experience pleasure often.   ☐ Yes   ☐ No

Occupational Self-Health and Solar Plexus Chakra

• I am confident of my skills, abilities and talents.   ☐ Yes   ☐ No

• I make my work enjoyable.   ☐ Yes   ☐ No

• My occupation and/or daily activities have meaning for me.   ☐ Yes   ☐ No

• I am taking action to insure my future financial security.   ☐ Yes   ☐ No

Relational Self-Health and Heart Chakra

• I spend meaningful time with close friends or family.   ☐ Yes   ☐ No

• I am able to forgive past hurts from others.   ☐ Yes   ☐ No

• I have at least one close friend and confidante.   ☐ Yes   ☐ No

• I love myself.   ☐ Yes   ☐ No

Self-Expressional Self-Health and Throat Chakra

• I communicate what I want and need to others easily.   ☐ Yes   ☐ No

• I speak the truth faithfully and speak up when I need to.   ☐ Yes   ☐ No

• I practice some form of creative expression.   ☐ Yes   ☐ No

• I am a good listener.   ☐ Yes   ☐ No

Mental Self-Health and Third Eye Chakra

• I avoid worrying.   ☐ Yes   ☐ No

• I am able to concentrate and focus when I need to.   ☐ Yes   ☐ No

• My problems provide opportunities for growth.   ☐ Yes   ☐ No

• I can visualize or imagine new possibilities as solutions to problems.   ☐ Yes   ☐ No

Spiritual Self-Health and Crown Chakra

• A presence greater than myself is always with me.	☐ Yes	☐ No
• My life has purpose and meaning.	☐ Yes	☐ No
• I meditate or practice quiet contemplation.	☐ Yes	☐ No
• I trust my intuition in making decisions and choices.	☐ Yes	☐ No

I responded No two or more times in the following dimensions:

_____

_____

_____

_____

Now, we'll start the process of attending to each of the chakras and the seven dimensions of self-health by covering each chakra in a subsequent chapter. If you can, imagine the chakras as energy centers, like the cylinders in your car. When all of your energy centers are firing fully, your life and your response to life runs easily. You feel fully powered, adaptive, responsive and effective. While it is no more important than any of the other dimensions, we will begin with PHYSICAL self-health and the BASE CHAKRA. The physical body is the most tangible aspect of our being and it will provide the most noticeable change in response to our actions in all energy centers.

As with this or any process of discovery in life, remember the wisdom of the turtle:

~ TURTLE WISDOM ~

~ Slow down

~ Be patient

~ Adapt to change

~ Be willing to stick your neck out

~ Know that you are always at home within your self

46

CHAPTER 6

HONOR YOUR BODY
~ The Art of Physical Self-Health and Balancing the Base Chakra ~

To bring forth the soul of our being, we must be in our bodies,
rooted to Earth, able to draw from the universal source of energy.

DIANE MARIECHILD

As a child and teenager I was always physically active. I loved to dance and actively play outside. I was sometimes considered a tomboy. I had particularly muscular legs, thunder thighs (as they were lovingly and teasingly referred to) and large calves that prevented me from wearing stylish knee-high boots (a big deal in the 60's and 70's). As I went through puberty, my breasts developed early and were a healthy size. I always felt larger overall than many of my girlfriends, thanks to my thighs and my breasts. I don't ever remember feeling attractive or sexy in a feminine sense, but I did feel the raging hormones and the desire for sexual experimentation with my steady boyfriend. The closest I came to really noticing and liking my body was when I was 15 and bought my first two-piece swimsuit. That "like affair" with my body didn't last long, because at age 16 I got pregnant after a brief time of sexual activity with my boyfriend. Boy, did that create an abrupt and unwelcome change in my body! Feeling comfortable with my feminine body quickly turned to shame. In 1970 teenagers rarely admitted they were sexually active and to get caught by getting pregnant was quite taboo! I became one of the girls who went away for months, harboring a secret. I hated losing the nice, athletic and feminine shape of my body, and I hated the ugly stretch marks on my skin. I hated having to hide my condition through a veil of lies, and I hated that I was having a baby when all my peers were having a good time! This experience created a detachment from my physical body for nearly 30 years. I came to fully accept, love and appreciate my body again during the process of training in The Nia Technique®. It was then that I was willing and able to fully immerse myself in the pleasure and wonder of my body, dancing freely while moving with sensuality, strength and awareness, and moving fully into appreciation of my powerful and flexible legs and my voluptuous and beautiful breasts. And to hell with the stretch marks!

48

*My body acceptance was challenged quite abruptly when I was diagnosed with breast cancer in 2006. My first reaction was, "How can my body be betraying me like this, when I have been so conscious about my health, especially for the last 7-10 years?" With the help of friends, family and healers, I soon realized that in order to move through the breast cancer treatment with renewed health, I must **trust** and love my body as a messenger with an innate ability to heal. Yes, my body was a trusted messenger of imbalance, unresolved grief, displaced guilt and over-nurturing others! It was important that I feel **safe and secure** in my body despite this clear signal of dis-ease. What I **did** know, and what I called on every day throughout my journey, was my daily rituals of connecting with my partner Bill and my continuing ability to walk in nature, dance, stretch, breathe and eat consciously. What I clearly needed to learn to do more of was "not doing," **relaxing** while allowing and trusting others to care for and support me. I have learned to **honor** my sacred body.*

The Art of *Physical* Self-Health in Everyday Living

Our physical body is both a sacred vessel and a wise messenger. Our body is the only vehicle we have for moving through life on earth. We can't trade it in for a new model like we do our cars. So if we expect to keep moving through life smoothly and for a long time, we better take care of our vehicle. Unfortunately, many of us don't pay much attention to our physical bodies. We spend so much time in our heads—thinking, planning, worrying, regretting, being inspired, creating and dreaming. Sometimes it seems that our bodies are just along for the ride. We have an over-active brain frantically leading our bodies around from one thought to another. We don't notice our body unless there is some message of discomfort. The *Art of Self-Health* invites you to seek, create and notice pleasure in your physical being, every day! The physical body provides wise feedback for your thoughts, emotions and actions. If you pay attention to how your body feels, it can tell you a lot about what you think, how you feel and how you act. Our physical well-being, vitality and resilience reflects the physical manifestation of the overall state of our being. The element of earth governs the physical body and the base chakra. Energetically, our physical body and the base chakra are about feeling safe and secure in the world. *The first place we need to feel safe is in our physical body!* If we can't feel safe and secure in our physical body, how can we feel safe in the world?

Love Your Body

One of the greatest challenges we must face on our journey to complete self-love and self-health is in loving our bodies. Societal messages about what constitutes physical beauty and attractiveness is pervasive and potentially harmful to the development of our compassion and love for our bodies. The aging process and the natural wear and tear process effects our physical appearance, agility and senses. Our skin loosens, our hair grays, our eyes need correction to see and our joints sometimes ache a bit. Well, this is your body, and your soul's vehicle. You've got to love what you've got because this is where you are now. You *can* positively change the function of your physical body with love and attention, but you can only start where you are *now* to become stronger and more agile, to create more energy, to lower your blood pressure, to relax your tense muscles, to reverse your diabetes, to build your immunity to colds and flu and to increase your flexibility to be able to touch your toes!

BODY SCAN MEDITATION

Take a moment now to sit comfortably, feet on the floor, legs uncrossed, arms and shoulders relaxed.
Close your eyes and take a couple of nice, slow, easy breaths. Then take some time to notice your physical body and any sensations present in your body at this moment. Start with your feet and toes. Move your awareness to your ankles and your calves. Notice your knees, your thighs and your hips. Move your awareness to your lower belly and your lower back. Notice the whole length of your spine, from your tail bone to the base of your skull. Notice your middle belly, your stomach, your ribs and your chest. Notice your shoulders and your neck. Move your attention to your arms, wrists and hands. What do you notice? Notice your throat, your jaw, your cheeks, your ears, your eyes, your forehead and your scalp. In any areas of your body where you notice sensation, simply notice, without judgment or trying to change. Have a gentle dialog or conversation with your body. Let your body know that you are listening and that you care. Now, move in front of a mirror. Look into the eyes of your SELF in the mirror. As you look into your eyes, honor all that has passed through you and all that you have experienced in your life. Honor the joys, honor the sadness, honor the love, honor the strength, honor the softness, honor the pain and honor the pleasure. Honor your SELF and the miracle of your body, exactly as it is.

50

The physical dimension of self-health is about honoring your body and creating a strong, safe and secure vessel for your earth walk. Physical self-health creates an adaptive and resilient container for the expression of the other six dimensions of our being (emotional, occupational, relational, self-expressional, mental and spiritual).

The physical body is a powerful messenger and it doesn't lie. Our body gives us signals and messages all the time, many of which we ignore or don't give credence to. *If we loved our self enough, we would listen to and pay attention to the messages of our physical body as often as we check our voice mail, text messages, social media or e-mail messages. In doing so we would receive the guidance we need for physical self-health.* Each of us responds differently to events of change, challenge, crisis, distress or demands in our life. Awareness of how you respond is important in consciously choosing to respond differently and to employ effective self-health tools to reduce the potential disease effects of stress. Below are common signals that indicate imbalance, but are often ignored. How many of these do you experience?

- ☐ Headaches
- ☐ Sleep disturbances
- ☐ Upset stomach/ intestinal disorders
- ☐ Clenched jaw
- ☐ Shoulder tension/tightness
- ☐ Clenched fists
- ☐ Short, shallow breathing
- ☐ Heart palpitations, rapid heart beat
- ☐ Cold, clammy hands
- ☐ Back or neck tension/pain
- ☐ Frequent crying
- ☐ Excessive eating/drinking
- ☐ Irritability
- ☐ Impatience
- ☐ Difficulty concentrating/ focusing on a task
- ☐ Poor productivity
- ☐ Difficulty making decisions
- ☐ Social withdrawal/inactivity
- ☐ Outbursts of anger
- ☐ Depression/ sense of hopelessness
- ☐ Low energy/lethargy
- ☐ Difficulty in relationships
- ☐ Constant worry
- ☐ Frequent colds/illness

All of these and many others, including common, preventable chronic diseases such as diabetes, heart disease and obesity, are our physical body's cry for attention. In our dis-ease our body is describing a lack of safety and security. It is saying "I am uneasy and having difficulty maintaining balance." Many of us live in a place of detachment from our physical body and its sensations, often as a result of a traumatic event or a deep physical or emotional wound. This could range from a childhood friend calling you "fatty" to traumatic sexual or physical abuse. It doesn't take much to disrupt the feeling of safety and security in our body.

There are five basic everyday components for supporting physical self-health and the base chakra. Each are equally important in balancing the energy of our base chakra. They are:

- Movement
- Nutrition
- Rest and relaxation
- Daily maintenance
- Care for your home

Movement

How we move our bodies is a reflection of how we move through life.

Our bodies are magnificently designed to ***move*** in all directions and in many ways. Movement is a powerful medicine. We are made for flexibility, mobility and strength. Yet the technology of modern life gives us every excuse to be sedentary and inactive. We can shop, prepare food, communicate and many times earn a living while sitting at a computer. Physical inactivity can indicate or perpetuate a state of stagnation or inertia in other aspects of life. Conversely, moving our bodies can be helpful in jump starting other positive life changes. For most people daily movement is not necessary for meeting basic life needs, yet it is widely documented that regular (at least 30 minutes a day) movement and exercise provides many life-enhancing benefits for both the body and the mind by:

- Reducing harmful stress hormones, such as cortisol
- Boosting the immune system and increasing resistance to dis-ease
- Lowering blood pressure, heart rate and respiration rate
- Stabilizing blood sugar levels to help prevent Type 2 diabetes
- Producing "feel good" hormones in the brain, such as dopamine, norepenephrine, serotonin and endorphins

- Increasing depth of breath, which feeds the cells with oxygen
- Increasing the ability to focus and stay on task

Start with the Breath

Breathing is movement. Our first breath as we enter this world is a deep, belly expanding breath! Watch a baby or a young child breathe and observe the easy rise and fall of the belly with each breath. Now, watch yourself breathe. What part of your body is moving with the breath? Your shoulders, chest, belly? Many of us typically begin to lock down our breathing and develop a habit of shallow chest breathing as a response to perceived stress. With this type of breathing the shoulders rise and fall with each breath and we are inefficiently using our body's skeletal moving muscles instead of our breathing muscle, the diaphragm. This can start when we are very young and begin to view our world as anything but perfectly safe and secure. Over time, short, shallow breathing becomes a habit, depriving our bodies of greatly needed supplies of oxygen!

Breath is the primary movement and life-giving force of our body, but if you pay attention, you may notice how often you don't breathe! Pay attention to how often you actually hold your breath throughout the day. Holding our breath is common when we are concentrating, or when we are anxious, upset or in pain. Breath is our most basic method for nourishing the body, moving energy and overcoming inertia, yet it is often the first bodily function that locks down. We will discuss more about breath when we address rest and relaxation, but you can begin now to expand movement in your life by simply practicing deep belly (diaphragmatic) breathing as outlined on the following page. This is probably the most important "tool" to include in your medicine bag for self-health. Deep abdominal breathing stimulates the vagus nerve, which increases the release of dopamine and produces relaxation. Deep breathing relaxes tight chest muscles and opens up blood vessels so your heart can beat more efficiently. It enhances creativity and energizes the body and the spirit, and it can be practiced anytime. Try it when you are driving, standing in line at the grocery store, watching your child's soccer game or a taking in the sight of a beautiful sunset.

THE CONSCIOUS BREATH

Take a Deep Breath

1. Lie on your back or sit comfortably in a chair with your feet flat on the floor.

2. Place one hand on your abdomen, just above your navel, and the other on your chest.

3. Breathe in slowly through your nose and try to feel your abdomen rising like a balloon filling with air. Your upper chest shouldn't move much at all.

4. Slowly exhale through your mouth with slightly pursed lips and imagine the balloon deflating.

5. Continue relaxed breathing in this way for 2-5 minutes.

6. Practice several times a day, even when standing in line or driving in traffic.

54

Belly Breathing

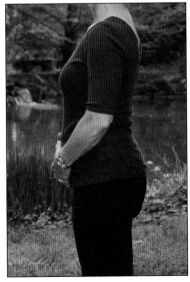

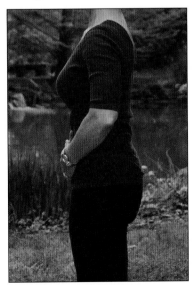

Inhale: Expanding lower belly   Exhale: Drawing lower belly in

Deep, mindful breathing can be practiced *anytime, anyplace, for any length of time*. Focus on the breath immediately brings your attention to your body and not only provides the body with nourishment, but also shifts the focus of the mind from the chaos out there to the calm within. When you can't control the situation out there, you can control your breath! Try it when you have a headache, are stuck in traffic, waiting in a long line at the grocery store, before an important phone call or meeting or when feeling anxious or foggy-headed. Move the breath and you move the stagnant energy.

After practicing this deep, relaxed breathing for a few moments, pause and notice how you feel, and note any new sensations in your body. Make note of those sensations here.

The Power of Movement: *Stretch, Strengthen and Energize*

Incorporating movement and exercise into our lives is both an art and a science. We need to create time and space in our daily schedule for exercise, and we need to find the type of exercise or activity that best fits our body's unique design and constitution and our unique emotional and mental cravings. Our stage of life, general health and even our social preferences can influence our choice of exercise forms. Are you best motivated when attending a class or do you prefer to exercise alone? Are you energized by music? For example, I teach classes in Pilates and movement classes based on The Nia Technique®. Over the years I have observed that the die hard Pilates class members are often different individuals than the dedicated expressive movement class members. People who gravitate toward Pilates tend to prefer structure, discipline and precision, while people who gravitate toward expressive movement prefer a more fluid and creative form of exercise. Personally, I love both forms, because I enjoy experiencing the extremes and the balance they each bring to my body/mind. Whole body fitness for physical resilience requires focused time and dedicated energy. The more we match our personal preferences and needs to the types of exercise we engage in, the easier it is to integrate movement into our everyday lifestyle. Whatever our choice, it is important to incorporate movement that nourishes our body/mind and provides a balance of *endurance, mobility* and *strength*.

The key ingredients to beginning, changing or expanding a movement regime in your life are:

- Start where you are.
- Keep it simple.
- Keep it enjoyable!

- **Endurance:** Cardiovascular and aerobic exercise is movement that sustains the heart beating at a rate that is sufficient for increasing its strength and efficiency (target heart rate). Your **target** heart rate is 60-80% of your maximum heart rate. It is recommended that individuals sustain a target heart rate for 10-30 minutes 3-5 times per week. Examples of exercises that can achieve a target heart rate and increase your endurance are: walking, swimming, cycling, dancing, walking the stairs, mowing the lawn with a push mower, tennis, racquetball, jogging/running, soccer, basketball.

To monitor your heart rate during exercise, find your target heart rate for cardiovascular exercise using the table below. Find the number closest to your age and follow the chart to determine if your heart rate is in the cardiovascular training range (60-80%.) For example, a 55 year old person would want a count of 17-22 heart beats during a 10 second count to be in a therapeutic range. *Always consult with your physician before beginning any exercise program.

Target Heart Rate
% of Maximum Heart Rate

AGE	55%	60%	70%	80%	85%
15	19	21	24	27	29
20	18	20	23	27	28
25	18	19	23	26	28
30	17	19	22	25	27
35	17	19	22	25	26
40	17	18	21	24	26
45	16	18	20	23	25
50	16	17	20	23	24
55	15	17	19	22	23
60	15	16	19	21	23
65	14	16	18	21	22
70	14	15	18	20	21

After exercising for 10 - 30 minutes, count your heartbeats for 10 seconds and find the corresponding number in the graph. This will indicate what percentage of your maximum heart rate you have reached.
Note: The pulse of your carotid artery can be felt and counted by placing your ring and middle fingers on the outside edge of your eye, then moving the fingers directly down your face to rest just under your chin.

One of my preferred forms of cardiovascular exercise is walking, particularly outside in natural surroundings. I realize that some days I am walking for my physical body, some days for my emotional and mental body and some days my walk is simply therapy for the soul! The pace and form of my walk changes each day, depending on the needs of my body, mind and spirit. Walks for the soul are definitely a little slower and more observant, both inward and outward, and walks for invigorating the body are definitely quicker and more energetic. Some of my greatest ideas, inspirations and healing visualizations come while I am walking. Following my breast surgery, I combined walking with "dancing" my arms and visualizing all of the cells in my body oxygenated, alive and vital. This movement provided not only medicine for my body—cardiovascular exercise and stretching the muscles of my chest and shoulders—but also medicine for my mind and spirit. I felt good from the inside out!

- **Mobility:** Stretching movement is overlooked and under performed by most people, yet it is extremely important in maintaining and increasing joint mobility and muscle flexibility. Performing at least 5–10 minutes of whole body stretching each day while incorporating deep, easy breathing can be both invigorating and relaxing. Movement forms that support the body's mobility are: yoga, Pilates and simple stretching while gently holding the position for 3-4 breaths. **Appendix A**, pages 138-146, includes specific moves for increasing whole body mobility and flexibility.

- **Strengthening:** Resistance exercise builds the strength of specific muscles while improving bone density and overall posture and health. Performing resistance exercise with weights, equipment, resistance bands or simply lifting one's own body weight (yoga, Pilates) 2-3 times a week benefits the bones and muscles and improves the performance of everyday activities involving pushing, pulling or lifting. **Appendix A**, pages 138-146, shows a few movements that use the body's own weight for resistance. No equipment needed.

When making a choice to add or increase the amount of movement in your life, it is more important to pay attention to how you *feel* during or after movement, rather than how you *look. If you feel good, you look good!* While exercising may be the last thing you want to do after a long day of work, it may be exactly the medicine you need to increase your energy and improve your sleep! While it is best to avoid active aerobic exercise the 2 hours before going to bed, slow gentle stretching may be a good choice to help you wind down from your day and relax before sleeping.

There are a number of holistic movement and fitness techniques that are worth exploring. They are: The Nia Technique®, yoga, Pilates, t'ai chi and various forms of martial arts (aikido, tae kwon doe). Any of these movement forms can energize, stretch and strengthen while also nourishing the mind, emotions and spirit. Many incorporate elements of relaxation, mental focus and individual expression with benefits for the whole being.

Nutrition

We are what we eat! What and how you eat affects how you think, feel and move. The food we ingest is the matter that we transform into energy. It provides support and nourishment for the renewal of our trillions of cells. Food is our body's fuel, just like gasoline or electricity is fuel for our cars. We wouldn't put watered-down or contaminated fuel into our cars and expect them to run efficiently. So how can we expect our bodies to run efficiently on heavily processed or "empty" foods, like sodas, candy, chips, donuts and cookies?

Individual nutritional needs are dependent on body type, lifestyle and activity levels. It would benefit your body and your base chakra to read and "digest" the information in a good book on nutrition. When making choices and changes to your nutritional habits it is also important to listen to your energy levels throughout the day to help determine what your body is asking for in terms of fuel.

Generally speaking, foods with minimal processing provide the best nutritional value. Eating more natural foods is not only good for your body, but can be good for the environment by eliminating the excess packaging for wrapping and boxing processed food.

While this is not designed to be a full course on nutrition, here are some basics about our primary energy source (food) and its benefits to whole health.

The Energy of Food

Different types of food fuel the body/mind in different ways. We all need some of each type.

Carbohydrates: Stimulate the release of **serotonin** which produces feelings of calm and peace. Complex carbohydrates are good sources of energy. What kinds are best? Complex carbohydrates of whole fruits, vegetables, beans, whole grains are high in fiber, which is necessary for effective elimination and cardiovascular health.

- *Vegetables:* Non-starchy and colorful are the best: broccoli, spinach, mushrooms, peppers, green beans, dark leafy greens.
- *Fruits:* Colorful and non-starchy are the best: apples, pears, oranges, blueberries, strawberries, grapes, kiwi, peaches, melons.
  ** Whole frozen fruits and vegetables carry much the same nutritional value as fresh.
- *Whole Grains:* Oats, millet, barley are also high in protein. Flaxseed is high in Omega 3 fats.
- *Limit and Avoid:* Sugar and white flour.

58

Proteins: Stimulate production of the neurotransmitter **dopamine**, which creates feelings of mental focus and concentration. High protein foods also help you feel full. ***Protein is the only nutrient that can build, maintain and repair our cells.*** What kinds are best?

- *Animal Sources:* Fish, poultry, lean meat, eggs, lowfat milk, yogurt, cottage cheese.
- *Vegetable Sources:* Peas, beans, lentils, nuts, seeds, soy milk, tofu.
- Eat some protein with every meal or snack each day.
- Including protein in your breakfast will help with mental focus and clarity.
- *Avoid or limit:* Red and processed meats.

Fats: Stimulate the release of **endorphins**, the body's natural opiate, and produce feelings of joy and happiness, **but only for a short term** (that's why people go back for more). Exercise, laughter and sex produce endorphins that last a lot longer! What kinds are best?

- *Monounsaturated and Omega-3:* Oily fish (salmon, herring, sardines, water-packed tuna), canola oil, walnuts, almonds, peanuts, soy products (tofu, soy nuts).
- *Healthy Heart Fats:* Olive oil, avocado, sesame, sunflower oil in small amounts. Daily fat consumption around 2 oz. (1/4 cup) is recommended.
- *Avoid:* Saturated fats (pies, pastries, cream, butter) and trans fats (hard margarine, fast foods, cakes)
- *Limit:* Hard cheeses (cheddar, parmesan).

Fluids: Keep the body hydrated and flush toxins. Drink eight glasses or cups of fluid each day, preferably water, fresh fruit juice or herbal teas. Sipping water throughout the day keeps hunger at bay.

Rest and Relaxation

Ah, the art of **NOT DOING**. We are a society which prides itself on doing more, having more, faster and faster! Many people operate in fight or flight mode (the body's overdrive stress response) all day, and drop into unconsciousness at night during sleep. We go from on to off without savoring the benefits of simply slowing down, relaxing and doing nothing. We have forgotten the art of simply BEING. After all, we are human beings, not human *doings*! Consciously bringing the body and mind into stillness gives our physical system a pause in activity, allowing us time to observe and feel the energy shift from overdrive to calm. And what a delightful feeling it can be! When we consistently allow the stress hormones and adrenalin to fuel our energy, we are stressing our organs and depleting our batteries or our energy reserves. In busy-ness we may feel energetic, but in reality we are operating on inauthentic energy, stress hormones. Our systems need a break! Conscious relaxation can slow our heart rate, lower our blood pressure, slow and deepen our respiration and calm our minds and emotions.

Incorporating relaxation into one's daily routine requires a conscious choice and it can be as simple as sitting and practicing deep belly breathing for a few moments. Other simple ways to consciously relax include sitting and watching nature (birds, butterflies, water/waves, a rain storm, deer grazing), listening to music, taking a bath, getting a massage, pedicure or manicure. Relaxation brings balance into our life by consciously nurturing our yin, pausing, to receive the calm, peace and beauty outside ourselves and within ourselves.

After living on the lake full-time for a couple of years, my husband Bill and I felt that we wanted to create a way to share the peaceful relaxation of the place with others, so we built Turtlecove Treehouse (www.turtlecovetreehouse.com) as a restful retreat and get-away surrounded by the nurturing sights and sounds of nature.

When we don't have guests, we will often retreat to the Treehouse ourselves for time alone or to reflect and focus. It has even been a great spot of inspiration for writing this book!

We all need a healthy dose of a quiet, restful retreat now and then!

60

Sleep provides our bodies with deep rest and stillness, which is critical for cell regeneration and energy restoration. Yet many people experience chronic sleep deprivation. Because of our high-paced lifestyles, we often do not get the amount of sleep we need, and accumulate a sleep debt. Our natural circadian rhythm (sleep/wake cycle) is disrupted. When people try to make up for the debt on the weekends, more imbalance and disruption of rhythms may occur.

Most adults need between 7.5 and 8.5 hours of uninterrupted sleep, yet many people discount the importance of sleep and pride themselves on being able to function with as little as four or five hours of sleep a night! Sleep is as important as food and air in supporting our health and vitality!

If you experience sleep disturbances, **Appendix C**, page 150, offers tips for better sleep.

Daily Maintenance

We all know that we can prolong the life of our car or home through regular maintenance. We can also increase the longevity of our physical body through regular attention and maintenance. It is important to enlist help to evaluate and support the health of your physical body. Regular maintenance and the *Art of Self-Health* means knowing your resources and consulting with conscious, holistic practitioners including, but not limited to medical doctors, dentists, chiropractors, physical therapists, movement instructors, naturopathic doctors, Chinese medicine practitioners and massage therapists. It is vitally important that we give personal attention and care to our skin, eyesight, hearing, and the health of our teeth, gums, bones, muscles and organs. Maintenance basics include much of what we have mentioned previously—eat well, drink lots of purified water, move your body, rest your body, floss your teeth, take in clean, fresh air, protect and care for your skin.

Care for Your Home

Yep, Dorothy (Wizard of Oz) had it right—*there is no place like home*, **if** you like your home. If you can't walk through the front door of your home and immediately feel good about where you are, then some change in your home environment may be in order. Just as our physical body is a place we must love and where we must feel safe and secure, so should our home environment be a place where we can feel at ease and slip into that comfy chair of our SELF. Maybe there are some rooms that you avoid going into, giving you a sense that you can't really live in your whole home. Pay attention to why that might be. Do you not like the color of the room? Is there too much clutter? Is there not enough comfortable furniture? Is there not enough light or too much light? Does the room smell funny? Are there uncomfortable memories in the room? Are there knickknacks or objects in the room that you don't like? Whatever it is, you can choose to change it. By creating your home space so you feel good, safe and comfortable you are putting energy into a very basic support structure and your base chakra. People who travel frequently, living in hotel rooms and unfamiliar places, often bring essential items from home, like their pillows, their favorite shower gel, family pictures, etc. to increase their comfort and feelings of home.

Energy follows attention! What you choose to give energy to (your physical self-health and your physical environment) will naturally expand in health, vitality and energy.

Basic Body Movements to Energize the Base Chakra

If you want or need to energize and balance the base chakra here are a few simple moves that can help.

Grounding: Stand comfortably with feet hip distance apart, arms at your side. *Inhale* and rise up on your toes, then *exhale* and come down firm on your heels, bending your knees slightly as you do. Pretend you are sinking into the floor. You may raise and lower your arms with the rise and fall of your body to emphasize and direct the energy down into the earth. Repeat this several times. Finally, stand quietly for a moment, knees slightly bent, breathing into your belly and bringing focus 2-3 inches below your belly button. Visualize roots growing from the soles of your feet deep into the earth.

Grounding

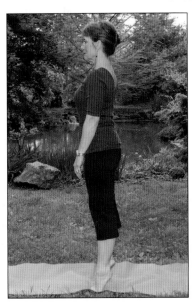 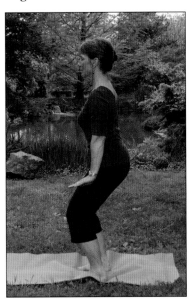

The Elephant: Stand with feet hip distance apart or wider. Bend forward with your knees slightly bent and touch your palms to the floor. *Modification:* Move your hands forward on the floor or rest them on your thighs or shins. *Inhale* and bend your knees about 45 degrees. *Exhale* and straighten your knees (almost straight, but not locked). Repeat until you feel shaking or a sensation of energy in your legs (usually within a few seconds). Keep your breathing full and relaxed during this exercise. Slowly come back up to standing upright. Shake your legs out, and stand comfortably for a moment, feeling the sensation of increased energy in the legs.

The Elephant

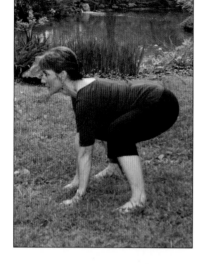 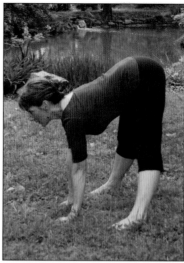

The Elephant *Modified*

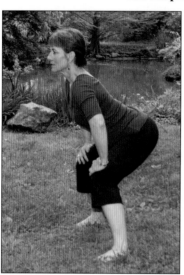 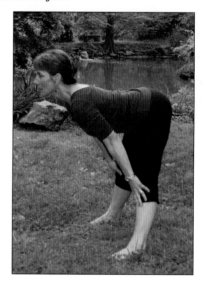

Push the Sky: Lie on your back and raise the soles of the feet to the ceiling with the knees slightly bent. Pull your toes toward your head and push your feet into the air, pushing through your heels. If you find a point where your legs are shaking or vibrating, stay there for a moment to energize your hips and legs. Notice the grounding sensation in your low back and sacrum.

Push the Sky

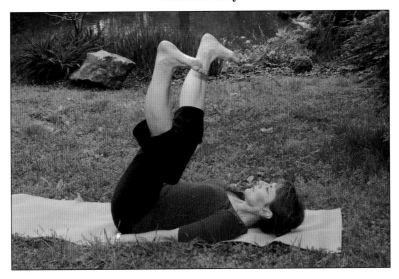

Mindful Walking, especially in nature, is a great way to nurture the base chakra. While walking, be conscious of your feet striking the ground and your breath in rhythm with your steps. Begin synchronizing the exhale breath to when a foot strikes the ground. This can be very grounding and bring increased awareness into your feet and legs.

Mindful Walking

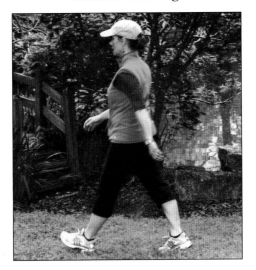

BASE CHAKRA
PHYSICAL SELF-HEALTH

Location: Base of the spine
Color: Red
Body parts: Lower lumbar and coccyx, feet, legs, bones, large intestines
Nature's Element: Earth
Archetype: Earth Mother
Personal Declaration: *"I Belong"*

SELF-ASSESSMENT

In Balance	**Mark the "in balance" characteristics that describe you NOW**
• Grounded	
• Feelings of safety and security	
• Strong immune system	
• Basic trust that needs are met	
• Good health	
• Good vitality and energy	
• Feelings of belonging	
• Comfortable home environment	
Out of Balance	**Mark the "out of balance" characteristics that describe you NOW**
• Fear about safety and security	
• Weight problems (underweight/overweight)	
• Frequent illness	
• Sluggish and tired	
• Problems with feet/knees/hips/base of spine	
• Sciatica (radiating pain in hip and leg)	
• Immune related disorder/Auto-immune disease	
• Uncomfortable home environment	
Self-Health Remedies	**What are you willing to do NOW to improve your Physical Self-Health?**
• Seek support (family, friends, community)	
• Listen to and honor my body	
• Practice deep, easy belly breathing	
• Move my body in ways that feel good	
• Eat tasteful, balanced, natural foods	
• Practice relaxation	
• Get adequate sleep (7-8 hours/night)	
• Create space, beauty and comfort in my home	

65

```
┌─────────── AFFIRMATIONS ───────────┐
│                                     │
│            for the Art of           │
│  Physical Self-Health and the Base Chakra │
│                                     │
│  I enjoy being in my body and I nourish it every day. │
│                                     │
│  I walk with my feet firmly on the ground, in trust │
│              and confidence.        │
│                                     │
│       "I feel safe and I belong"    │
│                                     │
└─────────────────────────────────────┘
```

Base Chakra and Physical Self-Health
Self-Reflection

- What is my physical energy level? Rate from 0-10, 0 being "I can't get out of bed" to 10 being "I have more than enough strength and energy to do anything I like."
- How have I honored the needs of my body today? (listened, stretched, walked, massaged, rested, healthful eating)
- How have I moved my body today? If I haven't, why not?
- How have I specifically moved energy into my base chakra today?
- What is my need for improved physical self-health?
- What is my **desire** for improved physical self-health?
- What **knowledge** and resources do *I have* that will support this desire? What knowledge and/or resources do *I need* to support this desire? What steps do I need to take to acquire the knowledge and resources?
- What is my plan for learning, mastering and integrating the **skill** that supports my desire?
- When I bring this skill into everyday **action**, how will it benefit me, my family, my community and the planet?
- What is most *enjoyable* about feeling good physically?

Self-Health Medicine Bag
Tools for Balancing the Base Chakra and Physical Self-Health

- **Move your body, and love your body** *every day.* Dance, walk, bike, garden, practice yoga, swim, etc.
- **Incorporate Everyday Moves to Stretch and Strengthen - Appendix A**, page 138, into your daily routine.
- **Practice Tips for Everyday Nutrition - Appendix B**, page 148.
- **Practice Tips for Better Sleep - Appendix C**, page 150.
- **Practice The Conscious Breath**, page 54.
- **Regularly check your body's messages** using the **Body Scan Meditation**, page 50.
- **Schedule and receive a massage.**

67

CHAPTER 7

ENJOY PLEASURE
The Art of Emotional Self-Health and Balancing the Sacral Chakra

We tend to think of the rational as a higher order, but it is the emotional that makes our lives. One often learns more from ten days of agony than from ten years of contentment.

MERLE SHAIN

*I had the good fortune to grow up in a loving and supportive family. My mother is very grounded, giving and compassionate. My father is a strong, smart and sensitive man, but has a loud roar. Dad was never one to keep his feelings of anger or frustration inside, and would verbally "blow off steam" and be done with it. I remember that the loudness of his anger made me uncomfortable, so I would often avoid situations of confrontation or making statements that might meet his disapproval whenever possible. As a result, for most of my life I experienced the expression of anger as expanding a feeling of "dis-ease" and discomfort rather than being a good thing. In my relationships with men over the years I have slowly learned that my partner's and my authentic expression of emotion—sadness, fear, anxiety, anger, joy, bliss—can create a healthy shift to pleasure and peacefulness in the relationship, IF communicated and moved from the inside-out in a healthy way. It has taken a lot of practice to allow myself to speak and move my own anger rather than holding it back in fear. It has taken practice to breathe deeply rather than tensing, crying or withdrawing when emotions are heated. My body is more relaxed and free to focus on **supporting** me rather than **protecting** me or **avoiding** situations. Today, I feel comfortable sharing my authentic emotions with my partner and my father... and I no longer take his loud expressions personally!*

The Art of *Emotional* Self-Health in Everyday Living

Our sacral chakra is the seat of our relating to others. It is the center of our needs, desires, emotions, sensations and our search for and movement toward pleasure. This energy center fuels our movement away from stability and security (base chakra) into dynamic interrelationships. It requires us to energetically move out in order to interrelate. This is the level where we begin to be conscious of and appreciate movement, change, adaptation and connecting with others. The element of water governs this energy center, bringing into our inner being flow and transformation. Water adapts to the outside element with which it has a relationship. When it flows onto a shore it seeps, trickles, rushes over, around, between and under the pebbles and rocks it meets. When water meets cold, it freezes and becomes rigid. When water meets warmth it melts and once again flows effortlessly. Water meets fire and it can boil or slowly expand and evaporate. The characteristics of water show up frequently in how we describe emotional responses, such as, "boiling with anger", "blowing off steam" or "giving an icy stare." Water also possesses a silky, soothing, sensual quality that brings a sense of pleasure and nurturance.

Our emotions are our body's way of teaching us about change and adaptation, and they can change at the drop of a hat. This usually occurs in our relationships to others, or our interpretation of an experience or event. For example, the way someone looks at you or says something to you can trigger a variety of emotional reactions, depending upon your relationship historically or at that moment in time. Some days your reaction may be anger, some days it may be happiness. Any relationship, whether it is with your parents, your children, your spouse, a friend or a co-worker requires constant adaptation. A mother may at one moment be playing happily with her children and in the next moment feel angry at her spouse for tracking mud into the living room. Or an employee may be feeling really bored and lethargic about his workload when his boss decides to give him an extra project that triggers feeling of excitement and renewed energy.

In this rapidly changing world, our ability to easily adapt and change helps overall resilience and our overall health. Individuals who can flow gracefully with changes in the financial market, job market, economy and even climate changes avoid unnecessary stress. Resistance to change causes self-imposed stress and tension. The more we can adapt to changes in people and circumstances around us, the healthier we

~ TURTLE WISDOM ~

When the shoreline is parched and hot, the turtle simply adapts to a different terrain. It easily changes its course from laboriously walking the scorched earth to buoyantly swimming the depths of the cool water.

are and the more enjoyable life can be.

Our emotions are dictated by our desire for pleasure. The word *emotion* (e-motion) denotes *energy (e) in motion*. Emotional self-health is supported by recognizing and acknowledging the need to move the energy of the feeling (the emotion) in a way that promotes and returns us to balance. When we emote, we are moving energy out of the unconscious, into the body and into the conscious mind. This cleanses the body, charges our energy system and promotes healing. Healing is any movement or change that creates a sense of greater well-being.

Anger, fear and joy all produce physical sensations. You can be "burning" with anger, "paralyzed" by fear and "full" of joy. Yet there are no bad or negative emotions. Some emotions may feel more or less comfortable than others, but all emotions are real and necessary messengers to *"do something, say something and move this energy!"* The key to emotional self-health is being honest with ourselves and others about emotions as they arise, gaining self-awareness and expressing emotions clearly, truthfully and authentically.

All emotions are real and authentic. Joy, bliss, peace, love and hope naturally produce feelings of pleasure and a desire for more of what feels good. Emotions such as anger, anxiety, fear, grief, hostility and frustration call on us to change a situation in order to restore balance and pleasure to our being. Unfortunately, many of us suppress or restrict full expression of the less pleasant emotions. This restricts both movement of the emotion and movement in the body by holding back, thus creating tension. Tension can be body tension (clenched jaw, stiff neck) or relationship tension ("you could cut the air between us with a knife"). It takes a lot of energy to suppress emotions. So expressing and releasing emotions (if done appropriately) releases tension. Releasing tension creates a harmonic, pleasurable flow within the body/mind while allowing deeper connections with others.

Thoughts, memories and experiences all carry an emotional component or charge that is integrated in our bodies on a molecular level and may unconsciously dictate our emotional response to life situations. Changing the programmed response requires conscious awareness and action. If you don't believe emotions carry energy, watch how the atmosphere of a room can change in response to a verbally loud, abusive or negative individual. Conversely watch the positive charge a room holds when occupied by people in loving, caring and peaceful relationship with each other!

Most of us are more comfortable sporting the body language of emotion rather than the verbal expression. Some of us avoid eye contact, cross our arms and clam up while others throw a whole body tantrum. Emotion is about relationship, with your self and others. This is most obvious when someone habitually triggers an emotional response in us. Pause here a moment. Can you think of a person or a situation that habitually

70

triggers an emotional response in you? Who or what is that? And what emotion is triggered?

Sexuality and Nurturance

Sexuality is a sacred life force and a ritual of union and relationship. It is the dance that balances, restores, reproduces and renews. Unfortunately, we live in a culture where we seldom celebrate the healthy expression of this element of our being. Our desire to seek the pleasure of our sexuality is viewed as self-indulgent or dirty rather than the expression of a basic life force that expands our energy and nurtures our relationship with our selves and others. Unfortunately, many individuals have experienced some degree of sexual abuse that casts shadows over the natural, loving nature of sexuality.

Denying the body intimacy and sexual release is denying our selves some of the greatest pleasure we can have. Denying this pleasure can cut us off from our wholeness, our sense of inner satisfaction and our peace. Sexuality is a movement of life, healer of the body and joiner of hearts. After all, we wouldn't be here without it!

If you are in an intimate relationship, talking about desires and needs with regard to sexuality can be a challenge. Yet sexuality is a natural life force energy that can promote healing on many levels, physically and emotionally. The more comfortable we are with our own sexuality, the more comfortable we can be in listening and sharing with the people who matter.

My pregnancy as a teenager caused a trauma of sorts to my sacral chakra and expression of my sexuality. It has only been in the last several years in my relationship with my husband that I have allowed myself to fully RECEIVE and experience not only sexual pleasure but also pleasure in everyday activities, like watching a sunset, savoring the taste of chocolate, letting my partner massage my feet, walking in a light rain or playing with our dog. Additionally I have learned to embrace sexuality as a way of nurturing myself and my partner. Enjoying pleasure every day, whether sexually or otherwise, is both nurturing and necessary!

Healthcare professionals and practitioners often use the healing power of nurturing and touch. Reaching out to touch, soothe and help others expands and feeds the sacral chakra energy of ourselves and the individuals with whom we connect. It is also important to be receptive to the nurturing that others give to us and create nurturance for ourselves. Receiving a hug can feel completely different than giving a hug. Yet both giving and receiving is vital for the harmony of our individual being and that of the planet. Nurturing ourselves is the first step in receiving or giving nurturance to others.

About four months after my breast surgery (a lumpectomy) I stood fully naked in front of a mirror looking at my whole body, my breasts particularly. I watched myself as I stretched my arms out to the side and over my head looking at the scar and the wound to my breast. There was a moment when I clearly saw and felt the energy of a warrior woman. I felt so sexy, so powerful, so soft and so beautiful! This was a woman whom I wanted to nurture! I stood there in acceptance of the changed physical structure of my body with full desire to nurture myself just as I am.

Anyone can nurture, and we all definitely need nurturing now and then. It feels good, produces feelings of peace, joy and pleasure, and sustains and renews our very being. Authentic emotional expression, sexuality and nurturance can all move us in an easy, flowing way towards a pleasurable relationship with ourselves, with others and a more peaceful existence in our world.

Basic Body Movements to Energize the Sacral Chakra

The Goddess Pose: This exercise puts you in touch with your sexual vulnerability. Lie flat on your back. Relax the hips and pelvis while bending your knees, bringing the feet close to the buttocks. Slowly allow your knees to part, while the soles of the feet come together. Allow the weight of the legs to gradually stretch the inner thighs. *Modification:* Place pillows under your knees to support the weight of the legs. Breathe slowly and deeply while holding this position for two minutes or more. Slowly and smoothly bring your knees together again. Then slowly open the legs while breathing in, and close the legs as you exhale.

72

Goddess Pose

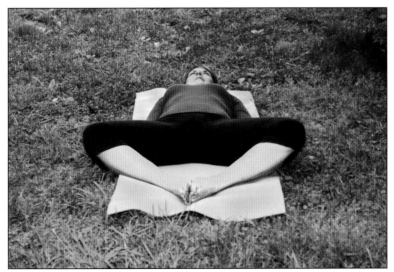

Pelvic Rock: Lie on your back with knees bent, feet flat on the floor hip distance apart. As you inhale, tilt your pelvis toward your pubic bone allowing the lower back to arch away from the floor. As you exhale tilt your pelvis toward your belly button so your low back is pushed into the floor.

Pelvic Rock

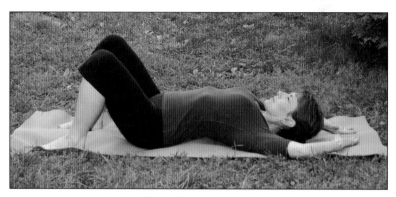

Arched Back (forward tilt of pelvis)

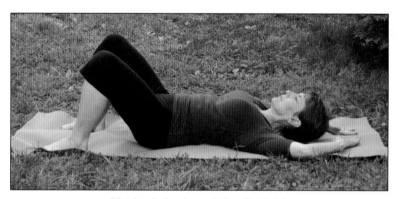

Flat back (backward tilt of pelvis)

Hip Circles: Stand with your knees bent slightly. Keeping the knees bent, begin to rotate the pelvis, creating circles with your hips. Begin with smaller circles, gradually increasing the circumference. Keep your head and feet in the same place and the movements as smooth as possible. Then rotate the pelvis in the opposite direction.

Hip Circles

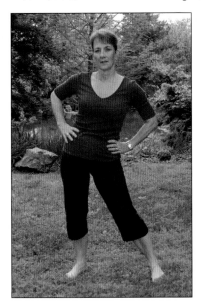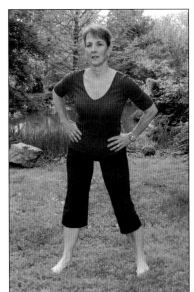

Hip Shakes and Swings: Stand with your feet hip distance apart, knees slightly bent. Begin shaking and vibrating the hips or swinging and dancing the hips. Keep the feet in the same place and play the arms overhead. Open your mouth and make fun vibrating sounds.

Hip Shakes

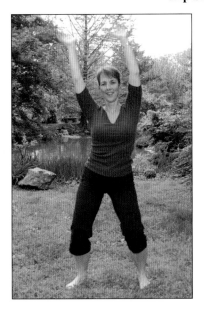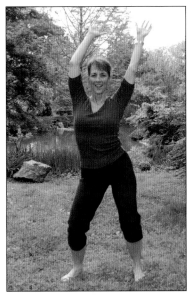

SACRAL CHAKRA
EMOTIONAL SELF-HEALTH

Location: Lower belly and low back between the navel and the pubic bone
Color: Orange
Body Parts: Sexual organs, genitals, bladder, lower abdomen, hips, groin, lower back, kidneys
Nature's Element: Water
Archetype: Lover
Personal Declaration: *"I Enjoy"*

SELF-ASSESSMENT

In Balance	Mark the Sacral Chakra "in balance" characteristics that describe you NOW
• Ability to experience pleasure	
• Healthy and authentic emotional expression	
• Ability to adapt and change	
• Nurturing of self and others	
• Graceful movement	
• Healthy sexuality	
Out of Balance	**Mark the Sacral Chakra "out of balance" characteristics that describe you NOW**
• Rigidity of body (stiffness/inflexibility) and attitudes	
• Controlling behaviors / Resistance to change	
• Denial of pleasure, sex, emotions, intimacy	
• Loss of appetite/passion for food, sex, life	
• Disorders of reproductive/urinary system	
• Sexual dysfunction	
• Low back pain/disorder	
Self-Health Remedies	**What are you willing to do NOW to improve your Emotional Self-Health?**
• Acknowledge desire for pleasure	
• Authentic expression of emotions verbally and through journal writing	
• Self-nurturance	
• Healthy boundaries in relationships	
• Watching, bathing and relaxing in water	
• Practice sacred sexuality	
• Practice letting go of control, stuff, need to know	
• Consciously embrace change	

75

AFFIRMATIONS

**for the Art of
Emotional Self-Health and the Sacral Chakra**

I make my decisions from a place of desire, joy and pleasure.

I flow with life in a graceful manner.

My sexuality is fulfilling and meaningful.

"I Enjoy"

Sacral Chakra and Emotional Self-Health
Self-Reflection

- How have I moved my body today, incorporating gracefulness and conscious breathing? If I haven't, why not?
- How have I experienced pleasure and nurtured myself today?
- What emotions do I find most difficult to express? Why?
- How can I be more emotionally authentic?
- How have I specifically moved energy into my sacral chakra today?
- How do I incorporate sensuality, sexuality and intimacy into daily life?
- What are my needs for improving my emotional self-health?
- What is my **desire** for improved emotional self-health?
- What **knowledge** and resources do *I have* that will support this desire? What knowledge and/or resources do *I need* to support this desire? What steps do I need to take to acquire the knowledge and resources?
- What is my plan for learning, mastering and integrating the **skill** that supports my desire?
- When I bring this skill into everyday **action**, how will it benefit me, my family, my community and the planet?
- What do I most *enjoy* about emotional self-health?

76

Self-Health Medicine Bag
Tools for Balancing the Sacral Chakra and Emotional Self-Health

- **Practice breathing.** Practice deep, rhythmic belly breathing. This can help to dispel rigidity and tightness associated with emotions such as fear, anxiety, anger and frustration. See **The Conscious Breath**, page 54.

- **Practice journal writing.** Begin to release your emotions to paper. "I feel…" is a good way to start the writing process and express emotions. This is also a good way to rehearse what you would like to say out loud. Studies have shown journal writing to be effective in decreasing pain and promoting healing in chronic illness or disease. See **Journal Writing - Appendix D**, page 152.

- **Practice self-nurturance.** Take a long, leisurely bath, get a massage, treat yourself to an afternoon, evening or weekend with close friends, give and receive warm hugs, sleep late, enjoy engaging in sacred sex or self-pleasuring.

- **Enjoy pleasurable body movement.** Put on some slow, sensual music and move your body in ways that feel good and make you feel sexy, sensuous, soft and fluid. Imagine your body as water, flowing with ease and pleasure. Observe and allow the breath to flow with the body.

- **Emote.** Put emotional energy in motion. Express purely and authentically how you feel. Move the emotions with the intention of creating and expanding pleasure and harmony. Verbally express using "I" statements. "I feel_____
when _____because_____.
I would like_____."

- **Practice intimacy and sacred sexuality** in your relationship. See **Suggestions for Enhancing Intimacy and Sex - Appendix E**, page 154.

CHAPTER 8

SHARE YOUR POWER

~ The Art of Occupational Self-Health and Balancing the Solar Plexus Chakra ~

Suppose you shine your ethical skin until it shines, but inside

there is no music, then what?

KABIR

For years I have been a closet writer. I have kept journal after journal of reflections, ideas, beliefs and inspirations, often thinking, "There's a lot of good stuff and life experience in here that might be of benefit to others." But I also thought, "Do I really have anything of value that people would want to read about?" My serious writing (which has really felt like playing) represents a willingness to step out and reveal my self in full form. The catalyst for writing this book was a clear message from my body. Prior to surgery (a lumpectomy) for breast cancer, I was told that an MRI showed what appeared to be a small metastasis of my breast cancer to my spine at T8-9 (on my back at the solar plexus). During meditation one morning I heard loud and clear, "You are holding back. What are you afraid of?" My answer was that if I wrote and published I could be read and recognized by thousands of people versus the hundreds that I am currently comfortable with. "This is blocked energy that you can clear by moving forward. You need to begin writing." I immediately realized that I had little to lose (other than cancer!) and I began the process of writing this book and putting my individual contribution out in the world in a much bigger way. I chose to step out of the shadows and let the light of the fire illuminate my gifts, talents and passion. And so it is. The energy that moves through our solar plexus has the potential to define our full presence, and our full presents…or gifts to the world. Epilogue: Ten months later the disease on my spine was reclassified and could not be differentiated from an old compression fracture. I truly believe that my writing was a step in taking full responsibility for my contribution to the health of the planet and my own health!

The Art of *Occupational* Self-Health in Everyday Living

When the third energy center, or solar plexus chakra, is in balance, it fuels the fullest expression of our unique gifts, talents and skills. How we choose to occupy our time, whether it is work that we get paid for, or leisure or volunteer activities is reflected in this dimension of living. We can choose how we expand a part of ourselves into the world in meaningful ways. How we do that helps generate a core sense of confidence, responsibility and self-esteem.

The yellow color and fire energy of this chakra represents the warm, powerful, transformational energy that is a natural manifestation of feeling strong and confident about our selves, our work in the world and our ability to contribute meaningfully to the whole of society. If how we choose to occupy our time is in alignment with our basic values, it is a more effortless endeavor to get up each day and feel good about what we are doing and how we are serving. If, on the other hand, we recognize that we are simply doing our job for the paycheck, it may be important to infuse these basic values into a hobby, volunteer endeavor or following a personal passion.

The saying "Work like you don't need the money" is about choosing work that you love, that sparks a passion and that has meaning. While money is certainly a necessity for meeting basic needs in life, meaningful work is a necessity for supporting occupational self-health and balancing the third chakra. ***Do you live to work, or do you work to live?***

Fire, the element of this center, takes fuel to burn. If we shut down, close ourselves off, criticize ourselves or withdraw from life, the fuel is deprived of the air it needs to burn, and eventually the fire is snuffed out. Only in a loving, dynamic state of interaction with the world, which requires getting out there and sharing our power and uniqueness, can we feed the fire that fuels our zest and passion for life.

~ TURTLE WISDOM ~
The turtle's shell makes it strong, but its **power** lies beneath its armor. Its ability to see and hear acutely is its unique gift, providing protection, self-responsibility and resilience by avoiding predators and staying the course.

Occupational self-health and the solar plexus chakra are supported by the full expression of our personal power. While much of society and the corporate world define power by titles, income, control and size, the personal power of occupational self-health is an inner power. This power comes from understanding and fully integrating *"I can"* be of value and *"I will"* take responsibility for my role on this earth walk. The fire of our personal power is fueled by our recognition of the unique spark of our individuality. We exercise our personal power by our willingness to share our individuality in ways that matter to us and to the collective whole of society.

Beginning the writing process has also exercised my *will*, overcoming the inertia of blocked energy that many times manifests as dis-ease. It mobilized my *desire* and accumulation of wellness-related *knowledge* and experience over the years. Exercising the will contributes to occupational self-health. Moving your gifts and talents into the world, in whatever fashion is a choice, and every choice we make is an act of will. You may catch yourself saying, *"I have to go to work,"* or *"I have to clean the house,"* or *"I have to plant my flower garden,"* when in reality you don't *have* to do any of this, but *choose* to do so because you like a paycheck and like to honor your agreements, or you like a clean house, or you enjoy flowers in the summer.

Balanced Responsibility

The fire in this energy center can easily dry up and burn out any juiciness (water) in our selves and in our relationships if we assume too much responsibility for that which is not ours. When giving attention to the solar plexus and occupational self-health, it is a good idea to revisit balancing yin and yang energies. In our occupational dimension, we can over-express our yang, or masculine energies by defining our worth and power by how much we do and how hard we work, and by taking too much responsibility for the happiness, success or financial security of others. A big part of embracing our individuality comes from becoming consciously clear on *how much* doing of *what* brings meaning and value into our own life. Burning your fire (solar plexus energy) just to make other people happy will soon lead to burnout. We are all responsible for our own happiness. If you take responsibility for your own life and your own actions, then the future and outcome are in your hands only, and your hands can be held loosely open, to receive the abundance that is yours for sharing with others.

Individuals full of power in their solar plexus exude warmth, relaxation and a vibrant sense of humor. The more confident you are in your personal expression, the easier it is to let go and laugh deep, healing belly laughs! Deep belly laughs and the breath that supports laughing are a great way to massage and fan the flame of the warm, fire energy of this third chakra.

Basic Body Movements to Energize the Solar Plexus Chakra

Power Walking or Jogging with Visualization: This quick forward movement provides intense, high-energy momentum that gets the blood pumping and the lungs breathing deeply. It is a great way to overcome inertia, particularly while visualizing intentions for self-health change. *See yourself "stepping into" the meaningful expression of your powerful self as you feel the energy running through your body, igniting the spark of positive change!* Periodically as you walk, stretch your arms and fingers out from the side of your body and up as far as you can, then slowly bring them back to your side, keeping them stretched and elongated. (Inhale as you raise the arms, exhale as you lower the arms.) Repeat this movement three or four times. The arms are the extension of ourselves that make contact with the outside world through our *creating and doing*. This movement activates the *outward* energy of the third chakra, moving the energy from the solar plexus and heart.

Power Walking or Jogging with Visualization

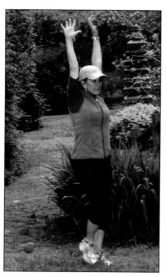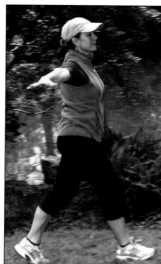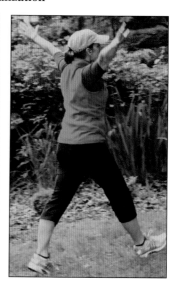

Back Plank: Sit on the floor with your legs extended straight in front of you and your palms on the ground behind your hips and under your shoulders. Squeeze your buttocks and lift your pelvis upward, creating a slight arch between your feet and your head. Focus on the solar plexus stretching and opening to the sky. Slowly relax and return to a seated position. Repeat two or three times.

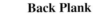

Back Plank

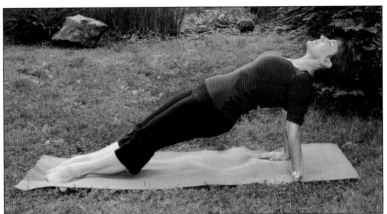

82

Belly Laugh Circle: This is a fun exercise done with at least three people, but the more the better! Everyone lies on the floor, each with his or her head on another's stomach. One person begins by saying a forceful "HA" three times, followed by the next person and the next. As your heads begin to bounce on the stomach below you, the circle breaks from "HA" into deep belly laughter!

Pike Pose: This one may be your challenge! Start by balancing on your tailbone while drawing the belly button in toward your spine. Lift your knees toward your chest and your feet off the floor while keeping your back straight. Slowly straighten the knees while keeping the torso up, creating a "V" shape with your body. Reach forward with the arms extending on the outside of the thighs. Hold this for three or four breaths, feeling the power in your solar plexus, then relax. This can be modified by lifting and straightening one leg at a time or keeping the knees bent while balancing and reaching forward with the arms.

Pike Pose

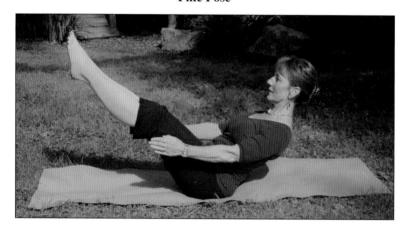

Pike Pose Modifications

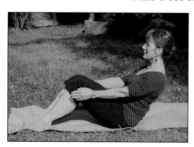 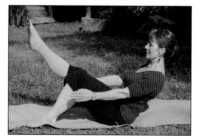

83

"YES" Dance: Put on some rhythmic music with powerful drums or percussion. While standing and without thinking, begin to create shapes with your body that are open, radiant, powerful and grounded. As you assume each expansive, creative shape, say "YES!" loudly and with full voice resonance. Feel the YES energy surge through your body and radiate out into the world! This is a powerful affirmation of your SELF and your creation in the moment. You might even feel silly and go into a belly laugh which is healthy too!

YES!

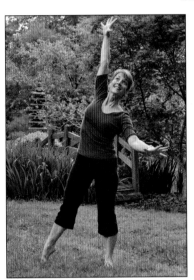 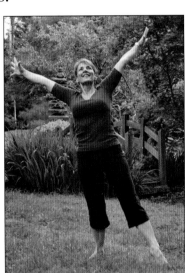

84

SOLAR PLEXUS CHAKRA
OCCUPATIONAL SELF-HEALTH

Location: Mid-belly / Mid-back
Color: Yellow
Body Parts: Digestive system, muscles, liver, pancreas, gall bladder
Nature's Element: Fire
Archetype: Hero
Personal Declaration: *"I Share"*

SELF-ASSESSMENT

In Balance	Mark the Solar Plexus Chakra "in balance" characteristics that describe you NOW
Confident	
Responsible and reliable	
Warm, spontaneous and playful	
Sense of one's personal power	
Sense of individuality	
Good self-esteem	
Satisfaction with chosen work and activities	
Out of Balance	**Mark the Solar Plexus Chakra "out of balance" characteristics that describe you NOW**
Irresponsible and unreliable	
Stubborn and competitive	
Low self-esteem/feelings of worthlessness	
Dominating or overly-dependent	
Low energy/chronic fatigue	
Eating disorders	
Diabetes or hypertension	
Job dissatisfaction	
Self-Health Remedies	**What are you willing to do NOW to improve your Occupational Self-Health?**
Acknowledge my unique gifts and talents	
Practice and share my unique gifts and talents	
Take responsibility for my SELF first	
Look for and find meaning in all I do	
Break inertia, get moving	
Strengthen my core muscles	
Plan for my financial security	
Practice spontaneity and play often	
Write a resume to "God"	

85

AFFIRMATIONS

for the Art of
Occupational Self-Health and the Solar Plexus Chakra

I honor myself and my unique talents and gifts.

I offer my light and service to the world.

"I Share"

Solar Plexus Chakra and Occupational Self-Health
Self-Reflection

- How have I moved my body today incorporating feelings of confidence, personal strength and power? If I haven't, why not?
- How have I specifically moved energy into my solar plexus chakra today (laughter, deep breathing, core strengthening)?
- When do I feel most confident and powerful?
- Which of my unique gifts or talents have I shared with the world today? What am I holding back?
- Can you imagine being excited to get up and do "your work" everyday? What would you be doing?
- What is my **desire** for improved occupational self-health?
- What **knowledge** and resources do *I have* that will support this desire? What knowledge and/or resources do *I need* to support this desire? What steps do I need to take to acquire the knowledge and resources?
- What is my plan for learning, mastering and integrating the **skill** that supports my desire?
- When I bring this skill into everyday **action**, how will it benefit me, my family, my community and the planet?
- What do I most *enjoy* about occupational self-health?

Self-Health Medicine Bag

Tools for Balancing the Solar Plexus Chakra and Occupational Self-Health

- **Break inertia and stagnation (light a fire under yourself).** Do something different. If you are sedentary, get moving. If you are always moving and doing, be still. Stretch and strengthen your core muscles. Drive a different route to work. Try scheduling routine activities at a different time of the day. Set the alarm for a different time each morning. Choose to do something that is challenging. Clear the clutter in your drawers or closets.

- **Lighten up!** Seek opportunities for a good belly laugh—watch a comedy, read a funny book, play games, spend time with funny friends; laugh at yourself and your silly goof-ups. Don't take yourself or life so seriously.

- **Take responsibility for what is yours only.** Acknowledge what you need and practice taking responsibility for your self and your happiness first.

- **Balance work values and well-being.** Use the worksheet in **Appendix F**, page 156, to identify what personal values are important to you and which ones are present in your work and everyday tasks. Make a plan for aligning your values with your work.

- **Complete your canvas of personal power** - **Appendix G**, page 158. Openly acknowledge your unique gifts and talents.

- **Write a resume to "God".**

CHAPTER 9

L O V E , L O V E , L O V E
~ The Art of Relational Self-Health and Balancing the Heart Chakra ~

This world is nothing but a school of love; our relationships with our husband or wife, our children and parents, with our friends and relatives are the university in which we are meant to learn what love and devotion truly are.

SWAMI MUKTANANDA

I believe that my diagnosis of breast cancer in April 2006 was a physical manifestation of my 'overtaxed' and out of balance heart chakra. The cancer manifested in my right breast, the side of the body that expresses yang or active energy. In the previous year I had experienced an immense amount of loss and grief as a result of my daughter's sudden death, my partner's stroke and the loss of my business and movement studio due to unexpected flooding. However, because of my habitual patterns of over responsibility, trying hard to please others and my "I can handle anything" mentality, I continued a fairly rigorous pace of teaching and supporting (nurturing) others through my work. Even though I felt that I was allowing myself to grieve and heal, my body obviously screamed otherwise, and clearly sent me a message I couldn't ignore—STOP, RECEIVE FROM OTHERS AND NURTURE YOURSELF! And pay attention, I did. It wasn't easy, but I slowly and consciously accepted myself and my physical vulnerability. I realized, despite the financial implications, that my most important job for the next year or so was to heal myself. And the first new belief I needed to integrate was that "self-health and self-love are NOT selfish!"

The Art of *Relational* Self-Health in Everyday Living

The element of air governs our heart center, providing energy that supports and guides us to be open-hearted and light-hearted, a necessity for optimal relational self-health. It is at the opening of the he*art* that the essence of the *Art of Self-Health* begins. Self-health begins with self-love and the relationship with SELF. The heart center is a gateway, which when open is like a swinging door on well oiled hinges. An open heart just as easily receives love as it gives love. We can actively love ourselves, but we must also be open to *receiving* the love we extend to ourselves. ***Self-love is not selfish!*** It is simply assuring that our cup is full before we extend it to others. If we only love, nourish and feed others, we are soon holding an empty cup and are living in a depleted state of loving. How can you give to others what you wouldn't give and receive for your SELF?

The fact that heart disease is the number one killer of both men and women in the United States points to the need for attention to this energy center and dimension of our well-being. We are having heart attacks, heart congestion, heart arrhythmias and heart blockages. All are symptoms, I believe, of not paying enough attention to the energies we are holding in our hearts (anger, resentment, grief, etc.) and not loving ourselves enough to really listen and act upon our heart's desires. The physical heart knows the importance of taking care of itself first. While its primary responsibility is to circulate oxygenated blood throughout the body, the heart first takes care of itself by nourishing the coronary (heart) arteries. Without this self-nourishment the heart would not be able to support the rest of the body.

The breasts and lungs are also governed by the heart chakra. I believe that the high incidence of breast cancer can be related to the over-nurturance (breasts) of others while leaving little for nurturing and loving one's self. Love and take care of your self first and there will be more available for others.

Extending unconditional love to your self and others means loving and extending compassion to the good, the bad and the ugly! Yes, there are undoubtedly parts of ourselves that are dark, shadowy parts that we don't like much. (I know very well an intolerant, judging, impatient tyrant that emerges from within me now and then.) But we can love our selves and extend compassion towards those less likable aspects of our being! Our SELF is the perfect practice ground for acceptance, forgiveness and compassion. When we embody and feel that for ourselves, it is so much easier to extend the same unconditionally and genuinely to others.

Exercising self-love is particularly challenging for women and healthcare professionals. We have adopted roles as caregivers. Much of our personal and professional life is spent literally reaching out and giving healing touch and attention to others. It is unfamiliar for us to relax and place ourselves on the receiving end of love and attention. While it may be unrealistic to make the shift to self-love overnight, it is a possible and a powerful shift to make.

Self-acceptance is the first step in practicing unconditional love. Start where you are. Love yourself as you are now, and feel compassion for *your SELF*. The more we love ourselves, the more love we have to extend to others. If all we do is give and give to others we are operating from a state of depletion rather than abundance. We must fill our own cup (receive love and nurturance ourselves) so that we have plenty to share! And the cycle of giving and receiving unconditional love begins and reciprocates ad infinitum.

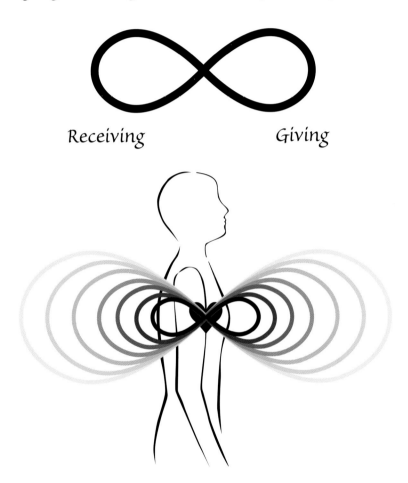

Receiving   Giving

The pulse of love from the heart center feeds the *Art of Self-Health* by weaving self-love into positive change in each dimension or chakra. For example, it is self-love that fuels the desire to create a new work schedule or environment (occupational self-health) that will provide a better match of our values or skills with our occupation. By creating this change we are feeding ourselves, filling our cup, so that we may continue extending love to others and ourselves! It energizes us to continue to make positive self-health choices. And the love continues to expand, on and on and on.

A healthy, loving relationship with self is the cornerstone for healthy relationships with others. When we love ourselves, we choose to surround ourselves with individuals who provide us with a healthy exchange of energy and continued nourishment. Take a moment to think of two or three significant individuals in your life.

When you think of the times you spend together, do you feel your energy expand (feelings of warmth, lightness, joy, peace) or do you feel your energy contract (cold, oppressive, negative or heavy feelings)? Expansive relationships generally provide a mutual and healthy exchange of respect, unconditional love, compassion and acceptance. They are life-giving and love-giving and they feel good! Relationships that produce feeling of contraction are often judgmental, critical, depressing and produce excessive neediness or negativity. The energy exchange is generally one directional and leaves you feeling like the life force energy has been sucked right out of you!

There are six of us in the "Yum-Yum" sisterhood. This circle of women friends magically formed through our common love of expressive dance. While we don't often get to dance together, our circle continues to gather and support one another, to this day. We are a diverse group of artists, corporate leaders, consultants, shamans, teachers, spiritual seekers, creators and dancers, who share a level of love, compassion and intimacy like no other group of friends I have known. We openly confess our deepest fears, our greatest joys and celebrations and our darkest moments, while laughing, crying and dreaming. Days before the surgery to remove my breast tumor, we sat in a circle on the floor in one woman's home, all of us baring our naked breasts in a show of love and support for not only me, but for each other, and all women in the world and their breasts. I shared with the group that I would like each of them to take turns blowing healing light into my breast with their right hand and then energetically extracting the unhealthy cells from my breast with their left hand. This amazing group of friends thought nothing of that request, thinking it not unusual at all, and went right to work! So the healing of my breasts and all breasts began lovingly and unconditionally.

In most cases we can choose with whom we spend time. Relational self-health is supported by loving your self enough to choose to spend time with and relate to individuals who are energy expanding. Choosing to limit time spent with individuals who contract your energy is also supportive of your well-being. Remember, you are responsible for your own happiness. Even energy expanding relationships can't make you happy, but *your choice* to spend more time with them can!

Relational self-health and the heart chakra is supported by freeing our hearts and love energy through forgiveness and healing unresolved grief, anger and resentment when appropriate. Loving your self enough to let go of these constrictive emotions will open the heart center, allowing the flowing and balanced interchange of giving and receiving love. Love yourself like a dog! Anyone who has had the life-enriching experience of receiving the unconditional love of a pet dog knows the kind of love that is joyous and limitless!

~ TURTLE WISDOM ~

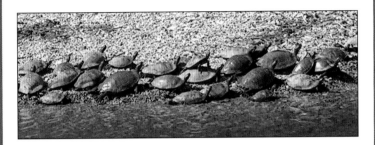

Turtles sun, rest and relax while
supporting each other with unconditional love.
They easily practice the art of both giving and receiving.

The unconditional love energy of this center nourishes, heals and sustains our physical being, but it also transcends physicality. Unlike the interchange of physical love expressed in sexuality, the love of the heart and relational self-health expands that which connects, nourishes and heals all people in the web of life. Love is the universal healer.

A Heart Broken Wide Open

Most of us have experienced a broken heart. Even though the healing can be painful, a broken heart often heals more widely open, leaving more space, expansion and air energy in the heart center. A broken heart healed wide open is more vulnerable, yet more open to give and receive the abundance of love available.

In 2000, I decided to take steps to find the son I had given up for adoption at the age of 17. I believe that my heart never healed from the grief of letting him go, although my head always knew that I did what I thought best for him, and his life's potential. I often felt that I was expected by my family and even some of my friends to just forget about it, and get on with life. I wasn't comfortable speaking about the experience, nor did I feel permission to grieve. As the years passed, my heart's desire to heal was calling more and more loudly. I needed to know after 30 years—is he alive, what was his life like, did I really do the right thing, does he have children, where is he living? And while I was excited with anticipation, I was also so afraid that he wouldn't want to have anything to do with me! A couple of months after I initiated the search, we did meet, and the healing began and continues today as we learn about each other and share some of our life experiences. It was that first courageous step that became one of many that opened my heart to a point of no return, gratefully! Not long after connecting with my birth son, my 20 year marriage ended, primarily because I was no longer willing to settle for living with a closed heart. Months later I met the love of my life, and learned pure, expansive, unconditional love for him when he had an unexpected stroke that affected his ability to organize in his brain and his ability to speak. Much of him changed before my very eyes, except his heart, which opened more fully to the exchange of our love. It was this love that sustained me when my daughter suddenly died. Again, my heart was broken wide open, yet I was loved and supported by an incredible community, and more open than ever to receiving the love. And I was going to grieve losing a child on my own terms this time! Much of that grieving was (and still is) done by talking about her and honoring her through unbridled expression of my love for her!

A few months after I moved to rural Oklahoma and to a more relaxed life living on a lake, I gathered one Saturday morning with a group of seven or eight women at the local YMCA. As we introduced ourselves we discovered that six of us had experienced the death of a child! What are the odds of that in a town of 6,000 people? I knew then that I was exactly where I should be, surrounded by compassionate women whose hearts had also been broken wide open! I simply said to them, "That's why we are here. So we can look into each other's eyes, give each other a hug, and say 'I know'." We had been given the perfect opportunity to show compassion for others, as well as for ourselves.

While the lesson of physical impermanence is woven deeply into my life, there is always a sense of permanence in the heart-centered love and compassion that I feel for myself, and for others who have experienced loss. I believe that it is the heart of compassion and love that will ultimately heal us and the world.

Basic Body Movements for the Heart Chakra and Relational Self-Health

Spread the Wings: Stand with feet hip distance apart. Reach straight forward with both arms, and bring the back of the hands together. With the inhale breath open the chest, bringing the arms behind the torso at shoulder level, opening the wrists by pulling the fingertips toward each other. Feel the stretch across the chest, shoulders and the entire length of the arms. Hold this for two or three full breaths, then on the exhale breath bring the arms forward with the back of the hands touching again. Relax the arms down at your sides and notice the sensations present.

Spread the Wings

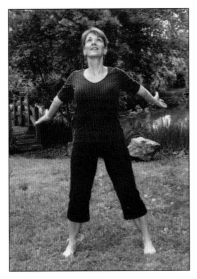 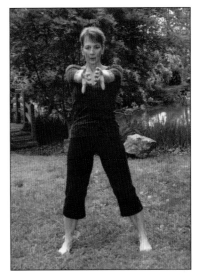

Inhale   Exhale

Windmill: Stand with feet slightly wider than shoulders. Stretch both arms out to the sides at shoulder level. Keeping the arms outstretched, rotate the torso back and forth while watching your hands pointing in different directions. *(Hands are the heart that touches the world.)*

Windmill

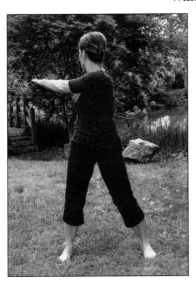 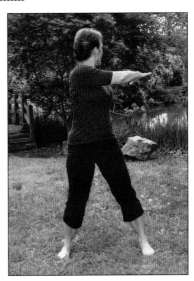

Exhale turn right - Inhale center - Exhale turn left

The Cobra: Lie flat on your stomach with arms bent and palms of the hands placed flat by your shoulders. Without using your hands or arms, slowly lift your head, shoulders and back as far as you comfortably can. Relax and lower the chest to the floor. Lift again going as far as you can without using the arms. Then use the arms and hands to push up a little farther, keeping the hips and pelvis on the floor without straightening the elbows completely. Hold for two or three complete breaths, then relax. Repeat as often as you like, noticing the opening sensation in the chest and abdomen.

The Cobra

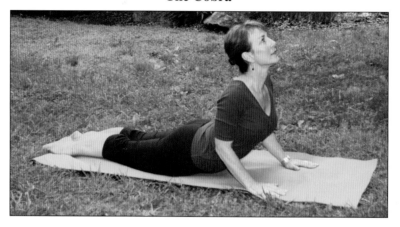

Modified Cobra

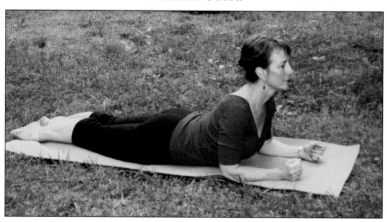

HEART CHAKRA
RELATIONAL SELF-HEALTH

Location: Between the breasts and shoulder blades
Color: Green
Body Parts: Heart, lungs, breasts, arms, hands
Nature's Element: Air
Archetype: Healer
Personal Declaration: *"I Love" / "I am Loved"*

SELF-ASSESSMENT

In Balance	Mark the Heart Chakra "in balance" characteristics that describe you NOW
• Self-loving	
• Loving	
• Compassionate	
• Empathetic	
• Forgiving	
• Altruistic	
• Peaceful	
• Joyous	
Out of Balance	**Mark the Heart Chakra "out of balance" characteristics that describe you NOW**
• Self-loathing	
• Resentful	
• Intolerant	
• Anti-social/withdrawn	
• Jealous	
• Co-dependent	
• Lack of compassion for self and others	
• Fear of intimacy	
• Disorders of lungs, breasts, heart, arms	
• Tension between the shoulder blades	
Self-Health Remedies	**What are you willing to do NOW to improve your Relational Self-Health?**
• Practice SELF love and nurturance	
• Practice forgiveness of myself and others	
• Seek to understand and practice compassion	
• Open my heart to receive love	
• Listen to my heart's desires	
• Nurture "energy-giving" relationships	
• Give and receive loving touch	

96

AFFIRMATIONS

for the Art of
Relational Self-Health and the Heart Chakra

I love and feel compassion for myself and others

unconditionally.

I openly receive love from my self and others.

"I love and I am loved"

Heart Chakra and Relational Self-Health
Self-Reflection

- How have I moved my body today incorporating feelings of expansion and lightness? If I haven't, why not?
- How have I consciously loved myself today?
- What "energy giving" relationships have I nourished today?
- How have I specifically focused on or moved energy into my heart chakra today?
- How have I expressed love to others today?
- How have I consciously received love today?
- To whom do I need to express more forgiveness, compassion and acceptance?
- What is my **desire** for improved relational self-health?
- What **knowledge** and resources do *I have* that will support this desire? What knowledge and/or resources do *I need* to support this desire? What steps do I need to take to acquire the knowledge and resources?
- What is my plan for learning, mastering and integrating the **skill** that supports my desire?
- When I bring this skill into everyday **action**, how will it benefit me, my family, my community and the planet?
- What do I most *enjoy* about relational self-health?
- How does relational self-health serve the greatest good of my being?

Self-Health Medicine Bag
Tools for Supporting the Heart Chakra and Relational Self-Health

- **Listen to your heart.** Take some quiet time to sit and check in with yourself. Listen to the guidance your heart provides you. After reading these words, close your eyes, take a deep, cleansing breath and say hello to your body and your being. Begin a gentle dialog. Are there ways you could begin treating yourself better? Are there parts of your body that are asking for nurturing attention? Do you treat yourself as well as you treat others? Are you as comfortable receiving love as you are giving love? Express gratitude to yourself and your body. What do you love most about yourself? When you feel complete with the messages received, thank yourself, open your eyes and write about what you heard.

- **Take a relationship inventory.** On a blank piece of paper write the names of individuals in your life that you spend significant time with. Write quickly as they come into your awareness. Now look at each name and notice how you feel as you remember the types of interchanges you have with that individual. Does your energy feel expanded (warm) or contracted (cold)? Circle or highlight those with whom you experience expanded energy. Cross out the names that generate a feeling of contracted energy. Now write an intention about creating a positive change in your relational self-health. Example: "I will schedule more time with _____and less time with _____" or "I will limit the amount of time I spend with _____to 10 minutes once a month".

- **Nurture every energy center (chakra) with the loving energy of your heart.** Practice the **Healing Pathways Meditation - Appendix H**, page 160.

- **Spend time in a loving, supportive community** such as a church or social group you enjoy.

- **Give yourself or your partner a loving massage *or* open yourself and your heart to receive a massage.** Imagine the loving energy of your heart center radiating from your heart through your hands, transmitting love with every stroke.

- **Write a love letter to your SELF.**

- **Reflect on ways that you could be more compassionate with yourself or others.** In what ways do you need to be more forgiving and tolerant of your self or others?

CHAPTER 10

EXPRESS YOURSELF
~ The Art of Self-Expressional Self-Health and Balancing the Throat Chakra ~

If you want the truth, I'll tell you the truth: Listen to the secret sound,
the real sound, which is inside you.

KABIR

For many years it has been my heart's desire to write a book and have the opportunity to speak publicly to groups about my passion, the relationship between movement and self-health. Until recently, my self-talk consisted of statements like "What I want to write has already been written in some form by others" or "I don't know how to write a book", etc. Until I changed my self-talk to "What I have to share is of value to others" and "I can only learn to write by sticking my neck out and doing it," this book continued to be a lump in my neck, literally. For many years I had a benign cyst on the back of my neck at the base of my skull and hairline (throat chakra). In the fall of 2008 it became large, red and angry, demanding to come out. To me it represented my words of wisdom that had been unexpressed for too long! Yes, our body talks to us in funny ways sometimes, and we can only understand if we listen.

The Art of *Self-Expressional* Self-Health in Everyday Living

Communication and creativity are the key components of Self-Expressional Self-Health. (That's a mouthful, isn't it?) So, if you can say "self-expressional self-health" three times without stumbling, you are in good shape! The throat chakra is the place of integration of the heart and mind. It is the energy center for sharing with the world our heart's desires and our imagination. This center carries our personal truth into the world through spoken or written words and the expression of our inner artisan, the creator. The throat chakra is governed by vibration, the energy that reverberates and sends waves of our soul into the world.

Through communication we connect, we teach, we share and we inspire. Through communication we share the song of our heart and the information in our minds.

You have no way to know what I am feeling, thinking or observing unless I somehow communicate it to you. Communication brings thoughts and ideas into manifestation. An idea for an invention only comes to fruition with a written description and perhaps a detailed drawing. A song only becomes a best-selling record when it is written and set to music. Unexpressed feelings, thoughts, ideas and beliefs are like putting a beautiful plant in a dark closet. We can't expect it to bring beauty and pleasure to us or others unless we bring it into the light.

If we don't communicate we have little or no relationship with the outer world. *How* we choose to communicate sets the tone of our relationships. Many of us have heard, "If you can't say anything nice, don't say anything at all." Yet communication—conscious communication—goes far beyond nice words. Words carry our desires and will into the world. Beginning sentences with "I feel," "I believe" or "I need" demands that you speak from your heart and from your truth in the best way you can. There is quite an energetic difference between saying "I'll *try*" and "I *will* do my best and see what happens." The language we choose to use can literally set the tone for our life experiences and for manifesting what we desire. Yelling, ranting, raging, using foul language and aggressive gestures invites others to put up walls and walk away instead of inviting constructive, creative engagement and dialog that supports our desires and will.

We all have unique skills, abilities and talents (solar plexus, occupational self-health), yet the world can only benefit if we communicate and express them. This energy center is perfectly positioned (in the throat) where the head and the heart often collide. You may have had the experience of wanting to say something tender or wise from your heart, when your head over-ruled ("you will be judged if you say that") so you end up with a huge lump in your throat or stumble all over your words!

The art of listening is also important to our self-expressional self-health. Listening and paying attention not only keeps us in synch with others, but also keeps us in synch with the world around us. Listening is a key component in any conversation. In fact, in many instances it is more important than speaking. Take a moment now and think of someone in your life that you consider a good listener. Now think about how you feel about that person. More than likely there are feelings of respect, caring, love or appreciation. I think we would all love to be considered in that same light. Are you listening?

Turtles may not have well-formed ears, but they listen well. They sit in silence and sense vibrations through their skin and shell. They "listen" to their environment by using their keen senses of smell and vision. Through the art and skill of listening they know when to act, hunt, protect and rest.

Tuning in to the sound of silence and listening to the subtle vibrations of the world around us, we can experience a more acute and rhythmic sense of timing and synchronicity in our actions. I have a wall clock that makes a soft, yet distinct, sound each second. When I sit, work or relax in that room my heart rate becomes "in synch" with the clock's 60 beats-per-minute rhythm. My body listens and absorbs the sound and rhythm even when my attention is elsewhere. My self-expression becomes focused, easy and productive. However, there are times when the rhythm of the clock feels too fast and I have to remove it or myself from the room to rest comfortably. When we surround ourselves with noise and chaos, even if we are not paying attention, our body will absorb that vibration on some level. For example, it is a lot easier to stay awake while driving at night if you are listening to up beat music or a talk show instead of slow, sleepy music. Being in synch with the rhythms of the world might show up in when you finally decide to make a major purchase and that particular item is on sale. Or it might show up when you call a friend at the precise moment they were picking up the phone to call you.

This energy center invites us to pay attention to our rhythm of living the personal vibration we imprint on the world. It asks us to assess whether our rhythm of living is in "right action." Is our rhythm of living natural and in alignment with what is good for us, our family, community and world? Self-expression moves energy outward in ways that represent our unique rhythms and our synchronicity with the rhythm of life.

For many years when I worked in the corporate world, I squeezed my self into its demands to work long hours, meet short deadlines, travel in the wee hours of the morning and hurry to meet all my obligations at home and at work. My level of burnout clearly told me that I was not in my optimum rhythm. Since my lifestyle has changed I can honestly say that "it hurts to hurry" now. I will if I have to, but it is an energy expenditure that I avoid when at all possible because it quickly triggers dis-ease and imbalance in my body/mind. My personal balance is worth getting up half an hour earlier so I can ease into my day rather than rush into my day.

I am especially passionate about one form of self-expression—teaching expressive, rhythmic movement and dance. I must, however, spend time listening to music before I actually lead a movement class or guided movement experience. Listening allows me to pay attention and internalize the unique rhythms, sounds, instruments and vocalizations which will guide my creative expression through my body. Only through listening am I able to understand, and through understanding, I can be a more creative and effective communicator of the art of movement.

A large group can easily become entrained to the voice and delivery rhythm of a speaker or presenter. One can feel the vibrant, electric and excitable energy that overcomes a whole room addressed by a loud, engaging charismatic speaker. Conversely, the peaceful calm of a room is palpable when a group is led in a meditation by someone with a soft, soothing voice. Oh, the power of vibration and the word!

Toning, singing and loud resonant voicing are techniques for moving the energy of vibration through the throat chakra, thus opening the pathway of self-expression. We all know the feeling of the lump in the throat or tightness in the neck and throat we experience before saying something difficult or self-revealing. Tears of emotion can easily be evoked by speaking our truth or by toning, singing or forcefully voicing. It is like opening the locked gate (throat) that has held under lock and key the emotions from the second, third and fourth chakras. This can feel very unsettling at first, yet can also be incredibly freeing for the body and soul!

Creativity

The sacral chakra (emotional self-health) is often seen as the energetic center of creativity because it is the center of sexuality and procreation. However, in the sacral center the *will* of the individual does not influence the detailed development and outcome of new life and whether or not fingers and toes develop perfectly in a new baby. In the throat chakra, however, it is our *will* that determines the outer expression of our hearts and minds. Through what we say, do, create and write we deliver our power into the world. The sound and vibration of our words and creations, even if spoken silently to ourselves, carry an energy force that can transform a feeling or a situation in an instant. A message delivered with patience and love carries a whole different vibration than one delivered with resentment or haste. Even our self-talk, such as "You will never be as smart as Tom," or "I feel fat and dumpy," creates the vibration of our being in the world.

I believe that many of us crave creativity and we don't even know it! I hear all the time from individuals in my workshops and retreats, "I don't have a creative bone in my body." We allow our life to be filled with the demands, desires and timetables of

103

others, leaving little or no time for SELF-expression. Creativity, like art, needs a blank canvas, or at least open space to be filled with our creation. In real life, this means that we must first clear out the clutter in our schedules, in our heads, in our living spaces, in our offices, in our cars, in our relationships, even in our spiritual practices, in order to have time and space for creation. Inspiration (in-spirit) is a source of creativity. The creation of our lives is a co-creation with Spirit—inspiration! Where do the ideas come from, anyway? When our lives are so full of clutter and busy-ness, we have no time to pause, listen and co-create.

Singing, dancing, writing, painting, gardening, cooking, photography, dressing style, re-arranging a room or a desktop or solving a problem on a work project are all forms of meaningful self-expression and creativity. Even designing the order of events in your day can be a form of creating! You are influencing your daily experience in accordance with your desires and preferences! That is why weekends and vacations that offer unstructured time are so important. They give us the opportunity to create and express ourselves in our own time and way. In every moment we have the opportunity to make creative and influential statements to the world through what we do and say and how we deliver those statements. Simple everyday ways to nurture your creativity may include:

- driving to work with a different route
- bringing something new and tasty for lunch
- wearing a bold new tie or scarf with a business suit
- rearranging your desk, your pantry or your living room
- not wearing a watch for a day
- engaging in a day of play with your kids
- sitting on the floor to sort files or pay your bills
- listening to music while working on a routine task
- taking a walk in nature
- using your imagination to create your perfect vacation or romantic rendezvous
- using a new herb or spice on fish, salad or roasted chicken
- not turning on the television
- brushing your teeth with your non-dominant hand or before your shower instead of after.

The possibilities are endless to express ourselves differently and creatively every day. When you incorporate something new in your life, share or communicate that new experience with someone. This is a good way to reinforce and further express the energy of the throat chakra.

Basic Body Movements for the Throat Chakra and Self-Expressional Self-Health

Head Lift: Lie flat on your back and relax. Slowly lift your head until you can see your feet, leaving your shoulders on the floor. Hold this position until you feel the energy move into your neck. This strengthens the neck and stimulates the thyroid gland.

Head Lift

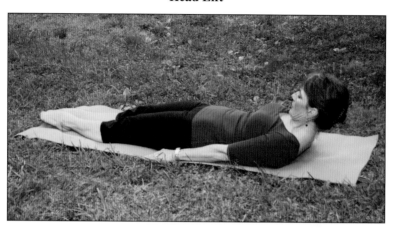

105

Neck Rolls: Sit or stand tall as if a string is pulling the crown of your head to the sky. Slowly roll your head in a circular motion. Pause at any point where you feel tension and massage that area of the neck with your fingers. As it relaxes some, move on. Move your head both clockwise and counter clockwise.

Neck Rolls

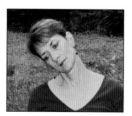 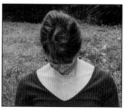 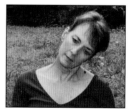

Fish Pose: Lie flat on your back. Slide your hands to the floor palms down slightly under the hips. Prop your body up on your elbows while lifting your chest towards the ceiling and opening the front of your neck until your head touches the floor. *Modification:* Place a pillow or bolster under your shoulder blades, then let your head fall back and open the chest. Hold for two or three complete breaths, then slowly lower the body flat to the floor.

Fish Pose

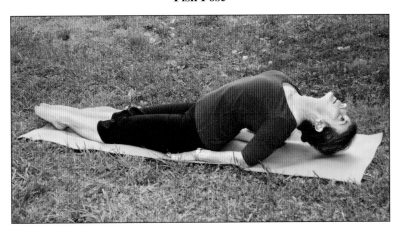

THROAT CHAKRA
SELF-EXPRESSIONAL SELF-HEALTH

Location: Throat / Neck
Color: Blue
Body Parts: Neck, ears, jaw, throat
Nature's Element: Sound
Archetype: Artist
Personal Declaration: *"I Will"*

SELF-ASSESSMENT

In Balance	Mark the Throat Chakra "in balance" characteristics that describe you NOW
• Clear, resonant voice	
• Good listener	
• Clear, open communication	
• Creative and expressive	
• Good sense of timing and rhythm	
• Positive language and self-talk	
Out of Balance	**Mark the Throat Chakra "out of balance" characteristics that describe you NOW**
• Introversion	
• Shyness	
• Too much talking and poor listening	
• Fear of speaking	
• Small, weak voice	
• Fear of trying something new or creative	
• Poor rhythm	
• Tightness of jaw, clenched teeth	
• Disorders of throat, neck, thyroid, ears, voice	
• Repetitive, negative self-talk	
Self-Health Remedies	**What are you willing to do NOW to improve your Self-Expressional Self-Health?**
• Practice singing and toning	
• Practice always speaking my truth	
• Ask for what I want and need	
• Practice being silent and listening	
• Try something new, practice creativity	
• Practice conscious language and self talk	
• Journal writing	
• Listen to beautiful music	

107

AFFIRMATIONS

for the Art of
Self-Expressional Self-Health and the Throat Chakra

I speak my truth with clarity and courage.

I sing the song of my heart in everyday activities

and encounters.

"I will"

Throat Chakra and Self-Expressional Self-Health
Self-Reflection

- How have I expressed my self creatively today? If I haven't, why not?
- How have I used my voice, vibration or movement to specifically move energy into my throat chakra today?
- In what ways do I tend to let my head overrule my heart resulting in miscommunication or false expression of my true self?
- How have I consciously listened to others and the rhythm of my world?
- What is my **desire** for improved self-expressional self-health?
- What **knowledge** and resources do *I have* that will support this desire? What knowledge and/or resources do *I need* to support this desire? What steps do I need to take to acquire the knowledge and resources?
- What is my plan for learning, mastering and integrating the **skill** that supports my desire?
- When I bring this skill into everyday **action**, how will it benefit me, my family, my community and the planet?
- What do I most *enjoy* about self-expressional self-health?

Self-Health Medicine Bag
Tools for Balancing the Throat Chakra and Self-Expressional Self-Health

- **Study and practice The Art of Communication - Appendix I**, page 164.
- **Practice journal writing.** See **Journal Writing - Appendix D**, page 152. Journal writing can also be an excellent "rehearsal" for saying out loud something that is difficult or emotionally charged. Practice writing what you want to say and how you want to say it while visualizing the person or situation in front of you.
- **Take a vow of silence.** Listening is an essential component of effective communication. When is the last time you consciously practiced silencing your voice for an extended period of time? By avoiding verbal communication we can open other avenues of communication such as writing, artistic creation, or tuning into the subtle vibrations of the universe. Begin with a few hours. Then try a whole day or longer.
- **Practice and acknowledge your creativity.** Make a list of the ways you creatively carry your uniqueness into the world. Open yourself to acknowledging your creativity at work, through parenting, at home, with friends etc. Set an intention to practice one or more of your creative acts each day.
- **Practice singing, chanting, toning.** In a room by yourself (or in your car) play some wordless, loud rhythmic music. After listening for a few minutes, begin to hum to the music. Then open your mouth, vocalize and follow the music with the tone of your voice while making vowel sounds such as "ah" "oh" "ee". When vocalizing, open your mouth to at least two finger widths between your front teeth. Allow emotions or tears to rise as needed. Listen to and feel the vibration of your own voice.
- **Practice only positive, life-affirming self-talk.** Practice awareness and notice the messages you communicate to your self. Talk to your self in the same way you would your best friend or lover. If you catch yourself making a negative remark to or about your self ("You dummy, you can't do anything right"), immediately say, "CANCEL/CLEAR" and rephrase the message in a positive manner ("I bet you could do better if you do it this way"). Each day take time to really look at yourself in the mirror and make a positive statement to your self ("You look happy today"). Remember, your body/mind absorbs the vibration of the expression and communication towards it.
- **Practice the *"YES!"* Dance.** See **Basic Body Movements for the Solar Plexus**, page 84.

CHAPTER 11

K N O W   Y O U R   W I S D O M
~ The Art of Mental Self-Health and Balancing the Third Eye Chakra ~

When the mind becomes quiet, you feel nourished.

SWAMI CHIDVILASANANDA

The world of reality has its limits; the world of imagination is boundless.

JEAN-JACQUES ROUSSEAU

Little did I know that a simple clinical in-service early in my occupational therapy career would be such an influential and life-saving experience. In 1979 I heard a presentation from Dr. O. Carl Simonton who was studying the effects of imagery and visualization in fighting cancer. He described how cancer patients were using the image of "Pac Man" (the big video game in the 70's) seeking and gobbling up threatening cancer cells in the body. His studies showed that this imagery was actually working to decrease the size of cancerous tumors. I distinctly remember having two thoughts at that moment: 1) "Wow! The mind really does have an effect on the body" and 2) "If I were ever to have cancer, this is what I would do to get rid of it!"

That single experience provided a launching pad for my own discovery, learning and eventual teaching of the mind/body connection. It also provided me with a tool that I later used in my own healing journey. However, being the peace-loving individual I am, I chose not to employ aggressive fighters or gobblers in my visualization. I chose instead to expand my loving, healthy cells to overcome the rebellious, renegade cancer cells (similar to using tough love with rebellious teenagers). Throughout my cancer treatment in 2006/2007 and even today, I daily visualize and feel as if my trillions of healthy cells are filled with light while supporting my strong, vital bones, organs, tissues and immune system. The light, vibrant, living cells are expansive and dominant when faced with any threat of dis-ease or imbalance. I simply focus on what I want to expand. Energy follows attention!

The Art of *Mental* Self-Health in Everyday Living

"Change your mind, change your world" is a good way to describe the power of mental self-health and the third eye (brow) chakra. Our reality is simply a reflection of our knowledge, perceptions and interpretations of life events. This energy center is fueled by how we choose to see the world and where we choose to give our attention. It is governed by light, and while we need light to see in our waking state, our third eye chakra also provides the energy that allows us to "see without looking." This is the center of our inner knowing and our intuition. *Energy follows attention.* What you choose to focus on will expand and become larger in your field of awareness. Even the process of choosing is a force of mental self-health.

Every tangible sensation and physical object in our world began with a thought or a vision. Think about it. You are surrounded by manifestations of the creative mind, yours and others. Even the chair you are sitting on began with a thought or a vision. At this very moment you are influencing the physicality of your body through your mind. How you interpret the concepts presented here creates an emotion, which creates a physical sensation and a physiological response. For example, if you perceive this book as helpful and relevant you may experience hope or optimism, which in turn could result in deeper breathing or a feeling of lightness. If you interpret these ideas and concepts as more to add to an already long list of things to do you may experience a feeling of frustration, resulting in a rapid heartbeat, tight jaw or muscle tension. Our mind, focus, interpretations and perceptions clearly have a direct influence on our physical and emotional well-being.

Try this simple exercise. Sit comfortably with your feet firmly on the floor. Close your eyes and take a few slow deep breaths. Notice how you feel, mentally, physically and emotionally and note any sensations in your body. Now think about a stressful event that you experienced in the last 24 hours. Place yourself in the situation, see the place and people involved, hear the conversation etc. Now, pause and again observe yourself. Notice any change in the sensations in your body—tension, gut reactions, heart rate, rate or depth of your breath, and write them here.

_____

_____

_____

For most people, the act of simply remembering a stressful event triggers the same emotion and physical response that occurred during the actual event. The change in how your body feels is the power of the mind influencing your emotions and your physical body. This happens in every waking moment. Just as you used visualizing in this exercise to negatively impact the body, you can also use it to have a positive impact. It is a matter of choice, of choosing where you focus.

Now sit comfortably with your feet firmly planted on the floor. Take 2-3 slow, deep breaths. Bring into awareness a pleasant memory, an experience that gave you a sense of peace, pleasure and joy. Place yourself in the time, place and situation with the people around you with whom you shared this pleasant time. See your surroundings, smell the aromas, hear the sounds and feel the air and environment. Now pause and observe yourself, noticing how you feel. Write down any changes you notice in your body.

_____

_____

_____

Wow. How quickly we can change our physical world by what we focus on!

Creating Calm from Chaos

Typically our minds are cluttered with an incessant stream of thoughts, many having nothing to do with the current moment. Much of our mental energy is spent worrying, or thinking about events of the past, or projecting ourselves into events of the future. We have no ability to change past events, and while we can use visualization to create a positive experience in future events, there is no guarantee there will even be a future. The only moment we can influence is NOW and how we choose to focus our minds NOW.

The present moment is filled with joy and happiness.

If you are attentive, you will see it.

THICH NHAT HANH

It is amazing how much stress we create in our bodies by where we give attention. Most worry is *fear*-laden and expands *anxiety*. Choosing to focus on the NOW, however, is an exercise of *self-love* and expands the sense of *peace*. The most effective way we have to shift our awareness from worry (past/future focus) to the present moment is to bring our awareness to our body. The sensations of the body provide a doorway to the present moment. Focus on the physical body is the perfect entry to the here and NOW. The most simple and healthful way to achieve that is through the breath. Practicing deep,

112

abdominal breathing (See The Conscious Breath, page 54) supports the health of the body, and clears the mind of "monkey chatter." This is a simple way to reinforce our awareness of the current moment. Mindfulness is exactly that, present moment awareness.

~ TURTLE WISDOM ~
Turtles are known for their longevity.
A turtle moves very slowly, somehow knowing that
it has all the time in the world.
Do we move quickly through life because we need to?
Or do we feel a need to because we perceive that there isn't
enough time?
Slow down and life will slow down with you.

113

Color and Light

The pineal gland is associated with the third eye chakra. Located in the geometric center of the head at approximately eye level, this gland serves as the body's light meter. It translates variations in light into hormonal messages relayed to the body through the autonomic nervous system. The autonomic nervous system is the brain/body function that controls unconscious bodily functions like heart rate, blood pressure, the size of the pupils in the eyes, skin temperature, etc. Many bodily functions, such as sleep and metabolism, have daily rhythms that are influenced by exposure to light. Think about how your body reacts and how your moods often change when daylight becomes shorter in the winter or longer in the summer. It is a natural tendency (as a result of our pineal gland and autonomic nervous system) to want to hibernate in the darkness of winter and grow things and play outdoors in the spring and summer.

Colors are the forms through which we perceive light. Colors carry definite emotional and mental effects. Red, for example is associated with initiatory or aggressive energies, yellow with hunger (note the color of many fast food restaurants), while blues and greens are associated with calm, peace and nurturance. Even light wavelengths beyond our visible spectrum have an effect on our health and state of mind. Fluorescent lights have been shown to have a negative influence on the health of plants and animals, whereas full sunlight, containing the complete light spectrum, has been shown to have a healing influence on arthritis, cancer and other diseases. One consequence is the "snowbird" phenomenon—older people, many with physical challenges, fleeing to areas plentiful with sunshine in the winter months. Interestingly, full spectrum light contains the full prism of light, the colors of a rainbow and the same colors associated with the chakras!

Visualization

Visualization is a powerful tool for creating the reality you desire. It is active dreaming. We all do it every day, all of the time, but not always consciously. While we are in the shower we may be visualizing what we will prepare for breakfast or what clothes we will put on. While we are working on a report, we may be visualizing how our supervisor will respond or how we will spend our time if we get it done early. Highly successful athletes visualize their body moving precisely and successfully going through the motions before the actual golf swing, bike ride, tennis stroke, swim event, etc. These everyday visions create our actions and our reality in the next moment. The more we visualize, the more vivid our mind's creations. Opportunities for practice are endless, and once it becomes a habit it develops naturally. The key is to be conscious of what you are seeing, believing and visualizing in ways that will best support a healthy reality.

For a couple of years after the death of my daughter I had a tendency to imagine and visualize the worst situation possible (death or disappearance) of my adult son anytime I didn't hear from him for a couple of weeks. I am not usually fatalistic, but I knew from experience that one's child could die unexpectedly. My imagination and visualizations were creating fear, tension and anxiety for me, and a hovering mom for a young man needing space, independence and trust. Finally, with the help of my son saying "Let go, Mom," I have let go of my fear and consciously shifted my mental energy to best supporting my son, and my SELF, by only visualizing his well-being as the outcome of his choices. I feel better, he feels better and our relationship is better.

On the other hand, during my journey through breast cancer, I was able to easily apply healing visualizations to my process and experience. During a four week period of time in April/May 2006 my supportive community and I used visualization to shrink the malignant tumor in my right breast from 2.5-3.0 centimeters (size determined by mammogram and sonogram) to 1.5 centimeters (size measured in surgical pathology report). The following is the specific visualization that I asked others to perform with me. "I visualize this area as simply a group of cells that is reluctant to come into perfect balance with the rest of my being. I see all of the trillions of other healthy, vibrant cells in my body, and particularly the healthy, vibrant cells in my breast, inviting the reluctant cells to transmute back into health and balance. If not, they will have to be removed and will not enjoy the blissful ride of my long life!"

I also asked for support in the following visualization during my surgery.

"I am safely and securely surrounded by a cocoon of intense and pure white healing light infused with love. This loving light supports the vitality and strength of my trillions of healthy cells while guiding the surgeon to perfectly remove all of the tumor and surrounding cells that are not supporting the whole vitality of my body, mind and spirit. (Some cancer cells may just dissipate in response to the light!) The energy center of my heart is softly, yet firmly supported by the many loving hands of my friends and family. (I see and feel the warm, open palms of support right between my shoulder blades on my back.)"

My surgeon read this visualization to her surgical team before starting the operation. She shared with me later that while the tumor was clearly defined, there was some tissue adjacent to it that "looked kind of like cappuccino." She said the pathologist in the room had never seen anything like it. They extracted the strange tissue, which turned out to be completely benign (non-cancerous). I shared with my surgeon that I believed the "cappuccino tissue" was simply cancer cells in transformation!

Beliefs

How we experience and interpret life events is closely related to our core beliefs. These beliefs are often learned and integrated into our lives through modeling or messages we receive from our parents, family, influential teachers, friends or by our own personal life experiences. They often govern our understanding of WHY things are as they are, or WHY we experience life events as we do. For example, if you have a core belief that life is always a struggle, or you have to work hard to have money or enjoyment, or you don't deserve money, health, or abundance, you will most likely find it difficult to attract or create work that you enjoy, that pays well and that feels effortless. On a more practical level, if you believe there is just not enough time in the day to do everything you want and need to, then you will have difficulty finding the time to care for your self-health, to prepare nutritious meals, exercise, meditate, etc. You will see and create what you believe. In turn, this determines what you focus on and give attention to, which in turn determines what takes up space and is most present in your life!

In 2008 I had finally had enough! Enough tragic loss and pain, enough disease, enough financial difficulty! While I had endured, survived and even thrived through major life changes in three years that many people don't experience in a lifetime, I was tired and craved to understand how I could shift from being what felt like a victim of circumstance to a co-creator of joy in my life! I wanted to know and understand some of the core beliefs that were shaping my experience of living. I wanted to live

115

authentically in joy and not wait for the next shoe to drop. So I sought help. I found a wise woman, intuitive guide and teacher who helped me see the impact of my core belief — "Whenever I take a risk and don't follow the rules, I get kicked in the butt!" *It became clear that this belief began when I broke the rules as a teenager, had sex with my boyfriend and got pregnant. Definitely what stood out then was the MISTAKE and the PUNISHMENT, not the pleasure of following a perfectly natural desire! Over the years, it became very easy for me to interpret challenging life events as PUNISHMENT. (I was a less than conventional parent and maybe didn't do enough for my daughter, so she died.) I came up against this same limiting core belief when I needed to make decisions about my post-cancer interventions. Consistent with my belief that "you see what you look for," I was not comfortable with having ongoing whole body scans to look for cancer that were not only costly, but exposed me to large doses of radiation. The rules of conventional medicine say one thing, and my belief system was saying another. My limiting core belief feared "if you don't follow the rules, your cancer will come back." So my belief needed to change. And I have consciously changed it. I will choose not to follow the rules instead focusing on and enhancing my health naturally, while avoiding insurmountable medical financial debt and the unhealthy stress associated with it. I will live each moment experiencing and deserving pleasure, joy and ease. I am choosing to assume full accountability for my choices. WOW! Do I feel free. This new awareness and conscious shift of belief and choice has returned to me a balance of pleasure, power and purpose.*

116

Basic Body Movements to Energize the Third Eye Chakra
Yogic Eye Exercises: This is a great exercise for strengthening and centering the eyes and is good for eyestrain, vision improvement and general fatigue from a lot of visual energy expenditure.

Begin in a comfortable seated meditative position with the spine straight. Close your eyes and bring your awareness to the point between your eyes, in the center of the head. Feel the darkness there and bask in the calm and quiet.

1) When you feel centered, open your eyes and gaze straight ahead. Slowly look upward as far as you can without moving your head. Then imagine drawing a straight line downward with your eyes, gazing as low as your vision can reach without moving your head. Repeat, return your eyes to center and close them.

2) Open your eyes again and center them. Then repeat the above movements, going from corner to corner, from upper right to

lower left, twice, and then from upper left to lower right twice. Close your eyes for a moment.

3) Open your eyes and repeat, this time moving from far right to far left. Repeat two times, then close your eyes.

4) Open your eyes and look "around the clock," first clockwise two times, and then counterclockwise two times. Close your eyes.

5) Keeping your eyes closed, rub your palms together briskly until you feel your hands become warm. Place your warm hands over your eyelids and let your eyes bask in the warmth and darkness. As the heat dissipates, slowly stroke your eyelids, forehead and face. Stop, open your eyes and notice how you feel.

Palming the Eyes

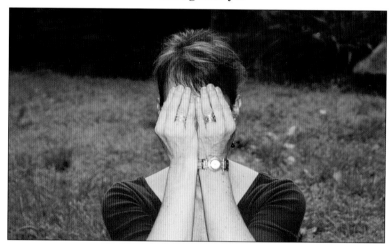

THIRD EYE CHAKRA
MENTAL SELF-HEALTH

Location: Center of the brow
Color: Indigo
Body Parts: Eyes, third eye, forehead, brow
Nature's Element: Light
Archetype: Seer
Personal Declaration: *"I Know"*

SELF-ASSESSMENT

In Balance	Mark the Third Eye Chakra "in balance" characteristics that describe you NOW
• Imaginative	
• Intuitive	
• Able to focus and concentrate	
• Perceptive	
• Good memory	
• Able to access dreams	
• Able to consciously visualize	
Out of Balance	**Mark the Third Eye Chakra "out of balance" characteristics that describe you NOW**
• Lack of imagination	
• Poor memory	
• "Tunnel" vision	
• Inability to remember dreams	
• Difficulty focusing or concentrating	
• Headaches	
• Problems with vision	
• Limiting beliefs	
Self-Health Remedies	**What are you willing to do NOW to improve your Mental Self-Health?**
• Revisit pleasant memories	
• Practice imagery or visualization	
• Witness and observe my thoughts	
• Examine my beliefs	
• Change my mind gracefully	
• Practice present moment awareness (NOW)	
• Use color therapy to enliven or calm (what I wear, color of my room)	

118

AFFIRMATIONS

**for the Art of
Mental Self-Health and the Third Eye Chakra**

I have a clear vision of all I desire.

In my stillness, I see all things clearly.

"I know"

Third Eye Chakra and Mental Self-Health
Self-Reflection

- How have I consciously used my memories, imagination or visualization to create positive feelings or experiences in my life today? If I haven't, why not?
- How am I aware of how I perceive or interpret life events and situations? Do I take time to witness my thoughts, emotions and actions?
- In what way to I notice my thoughts affecting my energy level and how my physical body feels?
- How have I specifically moved energy into my third eye chakra today?
- How and when have I consciously quieted my "monkey chatter" mind and focused on the present moment?
- What is my **desire** for improved mental self-health?
- What **knowledge** and resources do *I have* that will support this desire? What knowledge and/or resources do *I need* to support this desire? What steps do I need to take to acquire the knowledge and resources?
- What is my plan for learning, mastering and integrating the **skill** that supports my desire?
- When I bring this skill into everyday **action**, how will it benefit me, my family, my community and the planet?
- What do I most *enjoy* about mental self-health?

Imagination is more important than knowledge.

ALBERT EINSTEIN

Self-Health Medicine Bag
Tools for Balancing the Third Eye Chakra and Mental Self-Health

- **Focus on the moment and practice mindfulness.** Start by sitting comfortably and focusing on your breath. Notice the depth and rhythm of each breath. Notice the temperature of the air as it moves in and out of your nostrils. Notice the sensations in your body.
- **Notice your thoughts and the choices you make each day.** Awareness is the first step to making changes in your choices.
- **Practice A Guide for Visualization** - **Appendix J**, page 166, to create what you want in life.
- **Practice the color exercise** - **Appendix K**, page 168, to increase your awareness of how colors influence your life.
- **Examine limiting core beliefs** and practice turning limiting beliefs around to empower greater self-health - **Appendix L**, page 170.

CHAPTER 12

CONNECT

~ The Art of Spiritual Self-Health and Balancing the Crown Chakra ~

Spiritual power can be seen in a person's reverence for life…
hers and all others, including animals and nature, with a recognition of
a universal life force referred to by many as God.

VIRGINIA SATIR

*I opened The Movement Center in 2000 following a nine- month gestational period of dreaming, planning, building and financing. Little did I know that I was creating and giving birth to far more than a physical location with mind/body/spirit movement classes. I was giving birth to my own process of movement center, moving into my own center and remembering my own soul's purpose. I was not only creating a place where people could come to reconnect with themselves, I was creating a place where I would meet many of my soul's most kindred teachers and supporters along my path to self- discovery. The Movement Center was a catalyst for **my** movement center— into my comfy chair where I know my SELF best. When I arrived at The Movement Center to open up on a Friday morning in early December 2004 I found the entire space destroyed and flooded by a water line break. I felt as if the earth, my place of grounding had literally shifted under my feet. And while I had plans to move the center, it wasn't until January! The Nia community had just gathered the Saturday before to celebrate the space and bid farewell in a wildly emotional and energetic Nia Blast. One of my students and close friends said, "Carol, that space literally burst with all of the love and emotion contained there. It could hold it no longer. It was time to spread the love and let go!" The spirit of The Movement Center could no longer be contained in a place. It was a force of expanded love that needed to move forth into the world. This is also how I describe the appearance of my daughter as we shared dinner just hours before she died in a car accident. She appeared so bright, so light, and so full of spirit that her physical body could no longer contain the light. And it is this love and this spirit that supported me through the next few years of letting go, and letting go with love. My life was rapidly shifting and changing. But the one thing that didn't change was my inner being—my* *spirit, my soul, my essence, my love. My movement center was taking steps towards my comfy chair that is always there.*

Exactly one week after I let go of The Movement Center, I received a phone call that my partner, (not yet husband) Bill had had a stroke. As I watched him and supported him in his recovery over the next few months, it again became clear that the physical can be altered, but never the spirit and never unconditional love. In fact, I loved watching and feeling the heart of this strong, virile, independent guy expand gracefully in love, compassion and humility as he journeyed closer to his center of love. Even though he often had difficulty finding words to express his loving feelings due to aphasia, his eyes and heart were open and illuminated with love.

The physical can even totally disappear but the spirit remains. This image helped me tremendously in dealing with my daughter Courtney's physical absence when she died suddenly. I know that there is a part of her that is still here, even though her physical body has transitioned and disappeared. The love, the memories and the feelings of being connected to her are always present. Courtney affirmed this for me shortly after her death when she came to me in a dream. I asked her, "So Courtney, are you with God?" She said (in her usual indignant, yet loving way), "Mom, whether you say Spirit, God, Holy Spirit, it doesn't matter what you call it, it is right here (pointing to my heart). It is the essence of LOVE. That's what really matters!"

Indeed, the divine resides in our hearts, and is manifest as LOVE. Thank you, Courtney!

The Art of *Spiritual* Self-Health in Everyday Living

The art of spiritual self-health and balancing the crown chakra is finding purpose, meaning and the sense of divine intelligence running through all manifestation. It is our spirituality that gives form, focus and depth to all our activities. It is the why that supports our beliefs and activities. Spiritual self-health gives purpose and meaning to the choices we make every day. It provides us with a sense of connectedness to the whole of the universe. It is the essence of our being and the greater compass that guides the wisdom of the body, our ability to trust in a higher order, our beliefs and the awareness of a divine presence and oneness in all beings. Unlike the physical body, or the energetic emotional and mental body, this body of consciousness, our essence, is the core of our being that never changes. It is the part of self that is both small and still *and* infinitely expansive and connected to the matrix of all there is. The lotus flower in the center of the turtle model illustrates this concept. The thousand-petal lotus flower represents our infinite potential for expansion, growth and beauty. And just like the large violet center of the turtle, the spiritual dimension touches and influences every other dimension of our being. Our spirituality and spiritual awareness influence every part of our everyday being—*physical, emotional, occupational, relational, self-expressional and mental.*

Spiritual self-health is not about a rigorous religious belief or practice. However, the expression of one's beliefs through religion, ritual or community circles can provide a valid and meaningful platform for spiritual awareness and practice. If our chosen practice is one that expands our awareness, fills our heart with love, peace and joy, enhances trust in the perfection of divine order, and reveals the inherent light of our soul, then spiritual self-health is supported and expanded. Any practice that allows us to open further to life-giving information, possibilities and understanding expands the crown chakra and our spiritual self-health. Mindfulness meditation is one of the most powerful and effective practices for this. Sitting in stillness, objectively witnessing ineffective or unnecessary information and beliefs, allows us to be open to infinite life-giving possibilities.

Take a moment to stop, close your eyes and simply observe your breath moving in and out. Without trying to change anything, notice the rhythm, the depth and the temperature of the air as it moves in and out of your nostrils. **Who** is doing the observing here? Get in touch with the part of your being who is witnessing your body. Connect with the observer, that part of you that is never changing. This part of you is always quiet, centered, calm and without boundaries.

124

~ TURTLE WISDOM ~

In some cultures the turtle's shell represents heaven and the square underside is a symbol of earth. The turtle shows us how to unite heaven and earth within our own lives. It teaches us that we have the inner power to bring heaven to earth through our everyday thoughts, beliefs, feelings and actions.

I first began practicing daily meditation when my children were in their early teens. In our home the best place for me to sit in the mornings was in a loft area. It was up and away but not completely free from noise. I let my family know that I would be meditating at a certain time each morning and requested that they not disturb me unless absolutely necessary. During my meditation I was aware of my son and daughter getting ready for school, yet my focus and attention was on relaxing my body, allowing my breath to slow down and clearing my mind of thoughts. It actually was a great way to create a sense of peace for the whole household in the morning! My centered, restful alertness kept me present but detached from any chaos.

Learning to remain calm within the chaos is a great skill to have during these rapidly changing and challenging times and when raising children, especially as they move into their own transformative years as teenagers. Meditation is the art of doing nothing, connecting with that part of our self that is always peace and love. It allows us to tune out the outside world and cultivate the rich inner world. When is the last time you allowed yourself to DO NOTHING? Our culture prides itself on doing, accomplishing and achieving. Our bodies and minds are in a constant state of thinking, processing and activity guided by outside demands and influences. Meditation allows us to de-clutter, start fresh and recharge our mind battery. It also provides tremendous physiological benefits, such as increased oxygen intake, lower heart rate and lower blood pressure, giving the body/mind a deep rest while promoting a feeling of relaxation and inner peace.

Like any new skill, meditation takes practice. However, this spiritual exercise requires no special equipment, and simply taps into a state of mind that we know, but have forgotten or masked while navigating through our daily chaos. Studies show that meditation not only increases the levels of serotonin (a feel-good hormone) in the meditator's brain but also increases the release of serotonin in the brains of those in the same vicinity.

In Sanskrit, Hu – Man (human) translates into God – Being. Is it possible that we are beings expressing God though our human form? Rather than human beings having spiritual experiences, we are spiritual beings having a human experience. Our bodies, minds, emotions and even our personality can change every moment! Our bodies, our thoughts and our emotions are impermanent, yet there is a part of ours selves that never changes—our essence self, our soul or our divine self. This is really who we are. Imagine a house—the walls, the roof and the space inside. We can't really see the space inside but we know it is there, like our essence. Now imagine removing the roof and pulling down all the walls. Even though the walls are gone, the space is still there! Your essence never changes. Even when you gain or lose weight, are feeling sad, are working hard or playing hard, or are sick, your essence, or your divine self, never changes. The container may change, but not the *center, or essence*, of the container!

Any state of being, practice or activity that fills us with a sense of lightness, joy, wonder and peace can be considered a spiritual practice. At those times our soul sings and our inner light illuminates at its brightest! Time itself seems to stand still or have no relevance at all. It is love, self love in its purest form, the divine in a state of delight! It may be when we are sharing with a circle of friends, listening to inspirational music, watching the ocean waves, creating and planting a beautiful garden, sewing a story quilt, making love with our beloved, meditating or praying silently. These are times when we are connected with the heartbeat of our soul, and there is a sense of timelessness, with no attachment to outside circumstances. When our spirit is full it touches and infuses each dimension of our being with love, because we *are* love. Our physical, emotional, occupational, relational, self-expressional and mental dimensions all seek the support of our spiritual dimension, our inner light and the connection to our soul! Our movement center allows the lotus flower, right in the center of the turtle, to flourish and feed our resilience, our patience, our adaptability and our connection to our SELF, all through being love.

Illness, Dis-ease and Spirituality

Dis-ease, illness, accidents and crises are often natural catalysts for expanding an individual's spiritual self-health. There is nothing like a potentially life-threatening episode to trigger awareness of one's mortality and fuel a desire to pay attention to living. Facing one's own death or the death of a loved one often deepens the search for life's meaning and sharpens the awareness of how life is infused with precious and rich relationships and experiences. While wake up calls are often woven into life's tapestry, a catalytic episode is not necessary to further awaken our spiritual connections. We must simply be willing to look deeper within and ask ourselves "why" to embrace the process of self-discovery.

What we discover as we enhance our spiritual self-health is that our inside light, our essence, is always present. It is a warm, comfy chair that is always available to settle into, whether we are running a marathon, making love, sitting in meditation or easing into death. Learning and practicing mindfulness and meditation allows us to reconnect and become familiar with that still, quiet, comfortable place within. We can live a vibrant, meaningful life of joy, pleasure and self-discovery, knowing that the place of comfort and rest is only a short journey within.

Basic Body Movements for Crown Chakra and Spiritual Self-Health

Sit, simply sit, with the spine upright. Practice doing nothing. Observe your breath. Quiet the mind.

Sitting Meditation

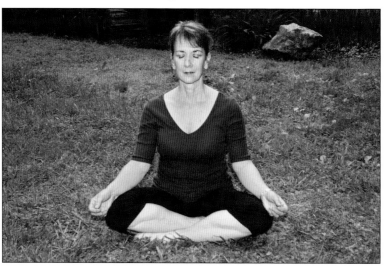

CROWN CHAKRA
SPIRITUAL SELF-HEALTH

Location: Crown of head and above head
Color: Violet
Body Parts: Central nervous system, cerebral cortex
Element: Thought
Archetype: Sage / Master
Personal Declaration: *"I Am"*

SELF-ASSESSMENT

In Balance	Mark the Crown Chakra "in balance" characteristics that describe you NOW
• Open-minded and aware	
• Thoughtful	
• Broad understanding	
• Wisdom	
• Able to question	
• Able to see larger pattern	
• Sense of spiritual connection	
• Trust "not knowing"	
Out of Balance	**Mark the Crown Chakra "out of balance" characteristics that describe you NOW**
• Apathy	
• Hopelessness	
• Difficulty learning	
• Rigid belief systems	
• Spiritual cynicism	
• Disassociation from the body	
• Over- intellectualization	
• Migraines	
• Brain disorders	
Self-Health Remedies	**What are you willing to do NOW to improve your Spiritual Self-Health?**
• Practice meditation	
• Pray	
• Spend time in nature/Connect with natural rhythms	
• Practice open- mindedness	
• Continue to learn	
• Practice gratitude everyday	

128

AFFIRMATIONS

for the Art of
Spiritual Self-Health and the Crown Chakra

I am guided by higher wisdom and divine love.

I find meaning, truth and purpose in all I am and do.

"I am"

Crown Chakra and Spiritual Self-Health
Self-Reflection

- How have I lovingly and consciously connected with my essence self today? If I haven't, why not?
- What is the higher meaning and purpose of my daily activities or work? Why am I doing what I am doing?
- In what ways have I been aware of universal rhythms and connectivity (nature or relationship experiences)?
- How have I specifically moved energy into my crown chakra today by quieting my body and mind?
- What is my **desire** for improved spiritual self-health?
- What **knowledge** and resources do *I have* that will support this desire? What knowledge and/or resources do *I need* to support this desire? What steps do I need to take to acquire the knowledge and resources?
- What is my plan for learning, mastering and integrating the **skill** that supports my desire?
- When I bring this skill into everyday **action**, how will it benefit me, my family, my community and the planet?
- What do I most *enjoy* about spiritual self-health?

Self-Health Medicine Bag
Tools to Support the Crown Chakra and Spiritual Self-Health

- **Spend time in nature.** Schedule and spend time in nature. Our natural world is a great teacher for living in a state of balance, trust and rhythmic wonder. Spend quiet time observing the ocean, a lake, or waterfall. Watch birds, listen to the trees in the wind, walk in a forest or garden. Breathe the fresh air, listen to the natural sounds surrounding you. Take a meditative walk outside, observing your being in the moment and the wonder of NOW. Reflect on your purpose in the universal whole.
- **Create ways to practice gratitude** - **Appendix M**, page 174.
- **Learn and practice meditation** - **Appendix N**, page 176.
- **Get comfortable with DOING NOTHING.** Practice sitting still and quiet for at least 10 minutes once a day.
- **Practice seeing and acknowledging the divine in every thing and every person.**

130

CHAPTER 13

ILLUMINE YOUR SELF
~ Enjoying Your Pleasure, Power and Purpose from Your Comfy Chair ~

The unexamined life is not worth living.

SOCRATES

I am often amazed at how my life habits have changed over the last 15 years and astonished when I remember the days when breakfast consisted of chocolate milk and a cigarette! I am grateful for my awakening, even if it met with occasional reluctance. Most changes occurred slowly by paying more attention and waking up to my everyday choices. In 1999, I didn't set out to write a book about self-health; I simply wanted to know more about myself. Although the overall process has been positive, there have been days, months and even years when I felt discouraged and derailed. Even now, in the depths of a cold winter's day, it takes a lot of mental and emotional energy and just plain tenacity to get out and walk 2-3 miles or get to yoga class. But even when I experience and accept a temporary lack of action or enthusiasm toward doing something good for my self I always seem to learn something.

Commitment to change takes determination and persistence. Most of us will fall into a dark hole and feel stuck at times during our process of change. Observe and be aware of your self. Solicit support, help and companionship from others. Enlisting a self-health buddy can be very beneficial in sticking with your process.

As we develop greater self-awareness and take steps towards greater life balance, remember, *the process is the outcome*. The key is to maintain a state of conscious awareness and mindfulness each moment of each day. Greater self-awareness provides both the process and the outcome. It does no good to worry about when we are going to be finished or when we are going to have all that we want integrated into our lives. Just having the desire to feel better and operate on full power will result in positive changes over time. Honor each part of the process as the outcome, for NOW. The chakras in full balance radiate the full spectrum of color, like a rainbow, and this rainbow represents the fully illuminated prism of our multi-dimensionality. Our light and our human (God-

Being) potential are infinite, and light will find its way through the smallest crack in the toughest exterior. Life's content and length are unpredictable, but how we experience our life is our choice. When faced with everyday challenges, choosing *discovery over despair* is how we grow and change. When we become aware of each energy center of our body and each dimension of our being, we bring that part of our being to light. Then we can examine, change and enhance that dimension of our SELF for our enJOYment.

Ah, yes. There is indeed considerable joy in easing into and resting in our SELF, into our comfy chair. Once we complete the journey of exploring the seven dimensions and the seven chakras, there is, if nothing else, a state of increased knowing, understanding and loving our SELF exactly where we are, how we are and who we are...NOW. Each day we have the opportunity to start where we are, with love, compassion and authentic desire. And because we know that we are always at home in our SELF, in our comfy chair, it is a great place to sit and honestly reflect, examine and dream. It is both a launching pad and a safe haven. It is home.

The nice thing about the pleasurable moments, weeks, or months of balance is that they teach us more clearly how uneasy imbalance feels. Desire for the comfort of balance serves as the impetus to seek greater personal harmony. But we can't get *too* comfortable, just comfortable enough with ourselves to ride with the changes. The good news is, once we experience balance, it always calls us back, and each time the journey is more familiar and less frightening. We will be familiar with our ability to navigate from a place of self-love with the backing and support of our comfy chair.

Light and the prism of color is a natural phenomenon. And maintaining our well-being should be a natural process. We have exactly what we need to return to balance and create our own *Art of Self-Health*. It simply requires that we pause long enough in our hectic lives to get back in touch with our SELF and allow *desire, knowledge, skill and action* to be guided not only by our inner wisdom, but by the tried and true practices of the ancients in eastern cultures and the way-showers in modern society. While our relatively young western culture would have us believe in the magic of medicating every symptom through prescribed pharmaceuticals, there is ample documentation of ancient and natural healing practices that have supported human beings for thousands of years. If we want a quick fix for dis-ease and imbalance, we can probably find a pill that will do the trick. But if we want a fix *and* a healthy dose of self-understanding and future prevention, then the journey inward is well worth the time and energy!

I chose a profession in allied health that most often provides rehabilitative services during a conventional medicine treatment and recovery regime. Occupational therapists play a large role in returning people to function *after* a health incident or crisis. While I recognize the value of conventional medicine, it is most often designed to treat

133

the symptoms and results of dis-ease rather than the cause. I believe that it is fully within our individual and collective power to understand and prevent the cause of our imbalance. While heredity can play a part in our susceptibility to certain dis-eases, we can enhance our immune system through healthful lifestyle practices. This decreases the chance of illness, but most importantly, it increases our resiliency and ability to heal from any dis-ease, imbalance or illness that does occur.

Creating self-health is an inside-out process. It requires enough self-love to:

~ TURTLE WISDOM ~
Be grounded and honor the body.
Adapt to change.
Share our uniqueness.
Seek support.
Be willing to stick our necks out and express.
Always be at home within ourselves.
Experience heaven on earth...NOW.

134

Personal transformation requires both toughness (the hard shell of a turtle) and soft vulnerability (the fleshy, inner core of a turtle's body). For the purpose of self-health, we are seeking to create a personal trinity of balance and equilibrium. We are bringing our body, mind and spirit in balance with pleasure, power and purpose. Love and self-love is the center for all relationships—the relationship of the body to pleasure, the relationship of the mind to power and the relationship of the spirit to purpose.

Creating balance requires staying grounded and remaining aware of our body sensations and its messages. It requires pulling inside to quiet and steady ourselves. It requires sticking our necks out now and then to explore and discover new, unfamiliar territory. It requires adapting to everyday changes and being patient and loving with ourselves in our change process. When necessary, we must be willing to connect with others and seek their support. We must embrace our inherent resilience, fueled by experiencing pleasure, power and purpose every day.

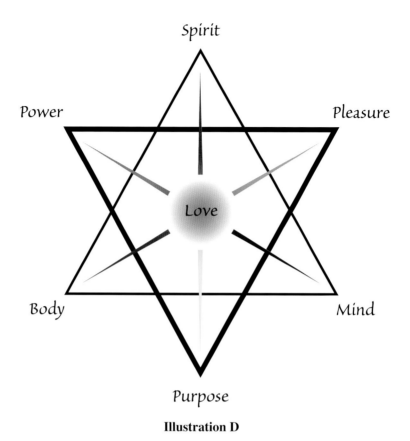

Illustration D

Illustration D illustrates the full spectrum illumination that occurs when love fuels and supports the interrelationship between body, mind, spirit and pleasure, power and purpose. *Pleasure* is in direct relationship to the *Body*. The body is the vessel for feeling good. It provides us with sensations of lightness, vibrancy and vitality. Our senses can be filled with pleasant sights, sounds, tastes, aromas, motion and touch and we can enjoy these when we are grounded in the body. Personal *Power* relates to that which we hold in our *Mind*. Our mind formulates and holds beliefs about our relationship with the world. The mind generates streams of creative thoughts and ideas, expressed as personal effectiveness through the clarity of vibration and truth. *Purpose* is the full expression of our *Spirit*. Our purpose of spirit represents our divine spark and is guided by our expanding level of responsibility, self-understanding and our sense of meaning and contribution to the whole. This relationship is demonstrated through the chosen actions of our lives. We can be a healthy, educated and spiritual person, but it all comes down to how we choose to live and express ourselves in the world, from the inside-out.

While I have spent well over 25 years seeking, learning and growing into greater balance, I recognize that I will never be "finished." Every opportunity or challenge that life presents or that I create serves as a call to greater awareness and expansion. The wisdom and everyday tools presented in this book are an accumulation of teachings, experiences and inspirations, for all of which I am extremely grateful. I also expect that I will continue to be open to my own expansion, simply by living in a more aware state of mind.

It is my hope that you will find your joy while creating your unique picture of self-health. The resources available to support your efforts are immense. **Appendix P**, page 180, provides a basic list of start where you are suggestions for activities and modalities that support each of the chakras and the *Art of Self-Health*. Be willing to stick your neck out and seek friends and qualified practitioners such as chiropractors, naturopathic physicians, nutritionists, personal trainers, yoga instructors, acupuncturists, reiki practioners, etc. who can assist you on your journey. But most of all, trust yourself and the power within to create the change you want to be.

It has become my daily ritual to wake up, look out over the lake and embrace the daily change of Mother Earth as reflected in the water, sky and woods. At the same time, I check in with my SELF—how can I best nourish my SELF today? Do I need to drink my cup of coffee in silence, watch the birds, write in my journal, talk with Bill, jump start my energy with a walk or yoga, or just get out into the world with my work of the day? I recently wrote in my journal that "I am feeling more and more comfortable with myself in this rural Oklahoma community." I realize that the peace that I feel is coming from me. I create my world by what I see, feel and do. I realize that many of my most rich and meaningful relationships are with individuals whom I've met while doing what I love and while being the most true to myself. I am feeling strong and clear about not having to please others or prove anything to anybody, including myself. I express my true self every day and there is a lot of freedom in that. Every day I commit myself to serving, working and finding joy everyday. My work in this world often feels effortless, yet meaningful. I trust that my basic needs will be met. My professional endeavors seem to have come full circle, as I am practicing more occupational therapy in traditional settings. Yet it is different. The full circle is a more expanded circle, because I am different. Through living with an attitude of discovery, I have grown and expanded. I know that every day there is opportunity for more joy and more expansion if I choose. I am at home with me. My energy is good and vital and I feel grounded and strong. I have compassion for my self during and through episodes of imbalance. I move and live at a pace and rhythm that allows for me time and time to invest in my loving relationships. My practice takes me to a lot of different settings, yet I find that I can easily adapt, usually with grace. I am confident in the value of my uniqueness in both new and familiar environments. I realize that I can create every day through the small things, and that there may be another book bubbling to be born. It is often a mindful ritual to wear my

136

favorite hat with the phrase "Life is good®" embroidered on the front and placed over my third eye. I know that my energy influences the energy around me. The sacredness of silence fills my soul as I commune daily with nature. I feel the inherent inter-connectedness of all living beings with the source of creation. In my comfy chair, in the deepest, most sacred part of my being, I am connected with that source. I realize that there is no right or wrong with life. It simply IS, each moment perfect for what it is. Self-love translates into energy and well-being, from the inside out.

Here is a suggested affirmation to consciously begin each day with your self-health in mind.

AFFIRMATION

Today I will listen to and honor the needs of my whole being...body, mind and spirit. I am willing to create time and space in my day to nurture my self-health in ways that expand my pleasure, power and purpose.

At the end of the day or after a self-health practice, offer gratitude to your SELF for bringing you closer to feeling more at home in your comfy chair of self-health. Here is a suggested affirmation of gratitude.

AFFIRMATION

I am grateful for and enjoy the renewable and resilient energy of my body, mind and spirit. I have abundant gratitude for all sources of inspiration and support, including my dedication to my well-being and the love for my self, moment by moment.

137

•
•
•
•
•
•

A P P E N D I X   A
~ Physical Self-Health and Base Chakra ~

Everyday Moves to Stretch and Strengthen

Whole Body Energy Wake Up: Inhale, arms open and overhead. Look up. Exhale and bend knees slightly and move tailbone and arms back (like wings), while looking straight ahead. Repeat 3-4 times.

Whole Body Energy Wake Up

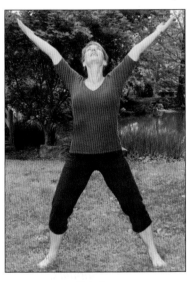
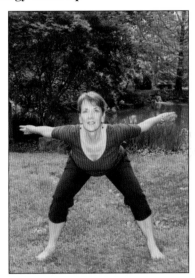

Inhale   Exhale

Spread the Wings Heart Opener: Inhale, open the front of the chest, bring arms behind, palms facing forward. Exhale, open the shoulder blades, and bring arms forward with the back of the hands touching. Repeat 3-4 times.

Spread the Wings

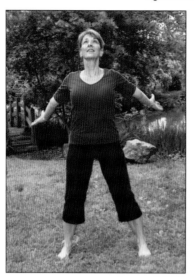 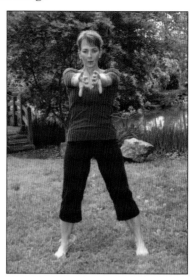

Inhale   Exhale

Modified Down Dog: Stand behind a chair with feet hip distance apart and hands on back of chair. Walk back until arms are straight. Keeping legs straight, lower the chest and reach back with the tail bone until the body forms an inverted L position and your head is between your arms. Hold this position for 4-5 complete breaths. Slowly return to standing position by walking forward and moving body upright.

Modified Down Dog

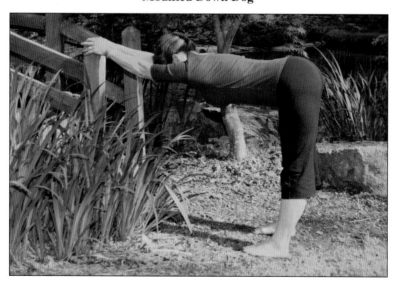

Sitting Spine Stretch: Sit on the edge of a chair with feet positioned slightly wider than hips. Place hands on thighs. Sit tall *as if a string was pulling the crown of the head toward the ceiling*. INHALE, look up and arch the back, opening the front of the body. EXHALE, lower the head, drawing the belly button in and round the spine into a C shape opening the back of the body. Repeat 4-5 times.

Sitting Spine Stretch

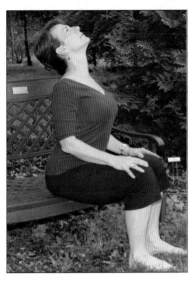 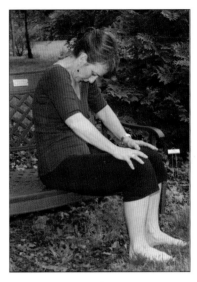

Inhale   Exhale

Sitting Hamstring Stretch: Sit on the edge of a chair with the spine straight and your feet hip distance apart. Straighten one leg forward, resting the heel on the floor with the toes lifted toward the ceiling. INHALE reach overhead with the arm on the same side. EXHALE while keeping head up and eyes looking forward, bending forward at the waist and reaching hand toward the toes. Rest the hand on the leg or foot while holding this position for 3-4 complete breaths. Notice the body's ability to move forward a little more with each EXHALE. Return to starting position and repeat with other leg.

Sitting Hamstring Stretch

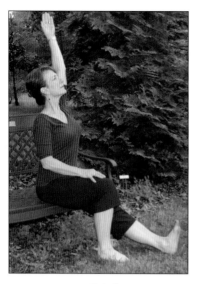 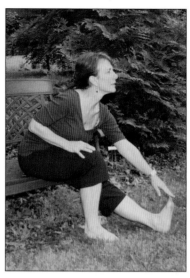

Inhale   Exhale

Seated Twist: Sit on the edge of a chair with the spine straight. Cross the right leg over the left. Place the left hand on the outside of the right thigh and right hand behind on the seat of the chair. Pull up through the crown of the head and turn the head and shoulders to the right to look over the right shoulder. Hold this position for 3-4 complete breaths. Repeat on the other side.

Seated Twist

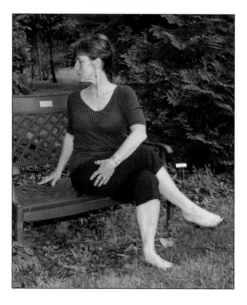

Seated Lunge with Arm Sweep: Sit on the edge of a chair. Turn toward the right. Keep the right buttocks on the chair. Step back with the left leg. Position right foot so the knee is bent no more than 90 degrees. You should be able to see the toes past the knee. Straighten the back leg while resting on the ball of the foot, heel lifted. Notice the sensation in the front of the left hip and thigh. HOLD for 2-3 complete breaths. INHALE, sweep the left arm forward and overhead, EXHALE move the arm behind and down, drawing a circle with the right arm. Repeat arm sweep for 3-4 breaths. ADVANCED move: Hold the leg position while lifting both arms overhead, looking up between the hands. Hold for 2-3 complete breaths. Return to forward sitting and repeat on the other side.

Seated Lunge with Arm Sweep

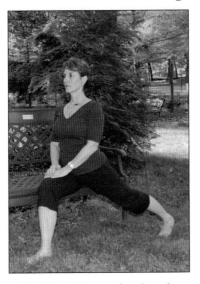
Hold for 2-3 complete breaths

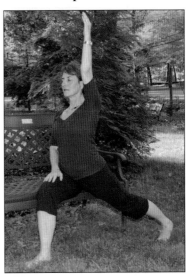
Inhale

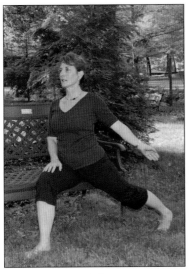
Exhale

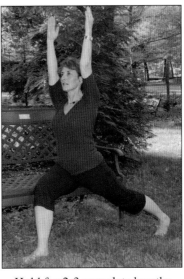
Hold for 2-3 complete breaths

Arm and Chest Stretch: Sit on the edge of a chair, spine straight. Interlace the fingers. Straighten and reach arms forward while turning the palms away. HOLD for 2-3 breaths. Keeping fingers interlaced reach the arms overhead with palms facing the ceiling. Drop the shoulders away from the ears. HOLD for 2-3 complete breaths.

Arms and Chest Stretch

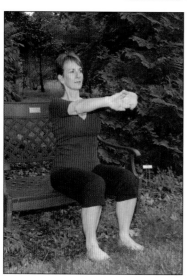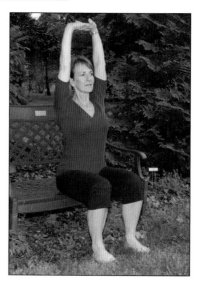

Supine Hamstring Stretch: Start on your back with knees bent, feet flat on floor hip distance apart. Bend right knee into the chest, hold leg behind the thigh or knee and straighten the knee. EXHALE draw the leg closer to you without bending the knee. HOLD for 1-2 complete breaths. *May add a "flex and point" of the foot while keeping the knee straight. Return to starting position and repeat with other leg.

Supine Hamstring Stretch

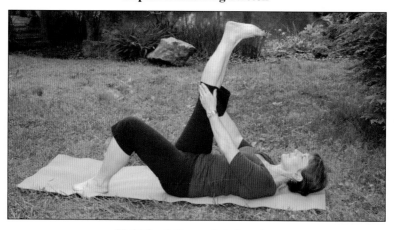

Hold for 1-2 complete breaths
Add "flex/point" of foot in this position

Extended Plank: Start in "all fours" position. Lift the right leg with a straight knee and hold parallel to the floor. Lift the left arm, straighten the elbow and reach forward with arm parallel to the floor. (Opposite arm and leg are lifted.) Position head, looking down and forward along the floor. Hold for 2-3 complete breaths. Repeat using the other arm and leg. *Strengthens shoulders, back, buttocks and hips.

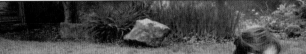

Extended Plank

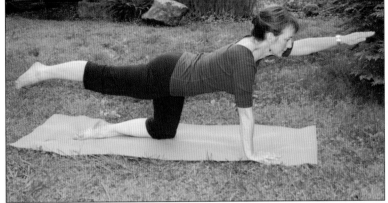

Swimming: Begin on your belly, arms extended overhead, legs close together. Lift head slightly to look forward. Keeping elbows and knees straight, INHALE lifting opposite arm and leg. EXHALE lower to starting position. INHALE lifting other arm and leg, EXHALE lower to starting position. Repeat lifting 3-4 times each side. *Strengthens shoulders, back (postural muscles), buttocks, legs, hips.

Swimming

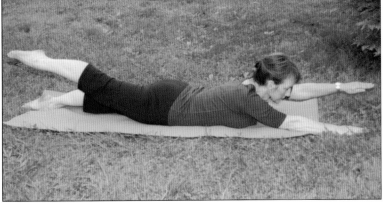

Bridge Pose: Begin on your back with the knees bent, feet positioned hip distance apart and arms at your side. INHALE and slowly lift hips up from floor, creating a "bridge" between the shoulders and feet. EXHALE and slowly lower spine to the floor one segment at a time until the back rests completely on the floor. Repeat 2-3 times. *Strengthens buttocks, hamstrings and back.

Bridge Pose

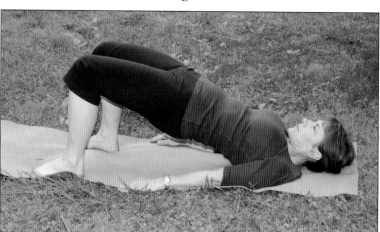

Reverse Plank Pose: Begin by sitting on the floor with legs straight in front. Place your hands behind your hips with fingers pointing to the side or toward your toes. Slowly begin to lift buttocks off the floor. Imagine reaching up to the sky with the belly and the chest. Look at the sky. Hold for 4-5 full breaths. *Strengthens the shoulders, back, buttocks and hamstrings.

Reverse Plank

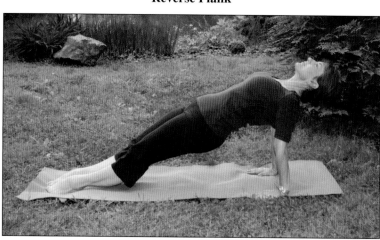

Pike Pose: Begin by sitting on the floor with your knees bent and feet flat on the floor. Slowly rock back onto your tail bone and lift your feet off the floor keeping your knees bent at first. Draw your belly button into the base of the spine to engage the core abdominal muscles. Slowly straighten the legs and reach the hands forward to the outside of the thighs. Hold for 4-5 complete breaths. *Strengthens the core abdominal muscles.

Pike Pose

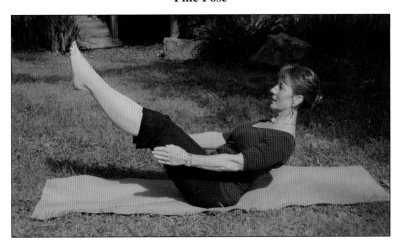

A P P E N D I X   B
~ Physical Self-Health and Base Chakra ~

Tips for Everyday Nutrition

Take time to stock up
- Fresh fruits and vegetables that don't need preparation: baby carrots, apples, pears, cauliflower, broccoli, grapes, strawberries, blueberries, etc.
- Whole seeds and grains for snacking: peanuts, walnuts, almonds, sunflower seeds, whole grain crackers
- Single containers of dairy: lowfat yogurt, lowfat milk, lowfat cottage cheese, lowfat string cheese
- Hard-boiled eggs for breakfast or lunch
- Pre-sliced and low sodium lean deli meats, canned tuna and salmon
- Take time on the weekends to prepare extra grilled chicken breasts, vegetable soup, salads etc. for weekday lunches
- Keep easy wholesome breakfast foods handy, such as single oatmeal packets, smoothie ingredients or protein drink mix, yogurt, eggs, whole grain breads, blueberries, bananas.

Find your unique healthy eating solution
- Try eating 5-6 small meals/day instead of 2-3 large meals and a snack. Be sure to include proteins and carbohydrates in each meal.
- Begin replacing fast food with healthy home food, one meal at a time. Then limit fast food to once every few weeks at the most, and be sure to be aware of the nutritional value of your favorite fast food.
- Increase your intake of fresh fruits and vegetables. Replace chips, candy or soda with these as your snack.
- Carry a healthy snack with you all the time. Almonds, sunflower seeds, air-popped popcorn, apples, grapes, carrots
- Practice taking *TIME* to eat away from your desk. Make eating a pleasant and enjoyable experience by going outside, visiting with a co-worker or friend. You will

find you slow down your eating and may even eat less!

- We are all different. Pay attention to how you feel and your energy level with different types of food.

Suggestions for "Quick Grab" Breakfast, Lunch and Snacks

- Single serving oatmeal
- Fresh fruit
- Hard-boiled eggs
- Whole wheat bagel / low fat cream cheese
- Low fat cottage cheese (mix with cut up veggies or fruit)
- Low fat yogurt
- Fresh vegetables with low fat dill or ranch dip
- String cheese and whole wheat crackers
- Water packed tuna and whole wheat or rice crackers
- Turkey or tuna sandwich on whole wheat bread
- Vegetable, chicken (skip the noodles)
- Grilled chicken breast, salmon
- Veggie burger on whole wheat bread
- Whole grain cereals (oatmeal, kashi, unsweetened granola with > 2 grams fiber). Add to yogurt
- Whole raw almonds, sunflower seeds, cashews
- Salad. Use balsamic vinegar and olive oil (sparingly) for dressing. Avoid bacon and croutons.
- Air-popped popcorn (no butter flavor)
- Water, herbal tea, green tea

HEALTHY SMOOTHIE RECIPE

Mix in Blender
1 cup low fat milk, juice, soymilk or almond milk
1 cup (2 servings) fresh or frozen fruit (blueberries, banana, strawberries, peaches, mango)
1 scoop whey or soy protein powder
2 tablespoons ground flaxseed

.
.
.
.
.
.
.

A P P E N D I X   C
~ Physical Self-Health and Base Chakra ~

Tips for Better Sleep

- **Pay attention to quantity and quality.** Most adults need between 7.5 and 8.5 hours of uninterrupted sleep. The need to press the snooze button in the morning may indicate that you are not getting enough sleep.
- **Keep regular sleep/wake hours.** Go to bed at the same time and get up at the same time every day. Getting up at the same time is most important. In the winter months it may also help to put a light (with a full spectrum bulb) on a timer to come on about the same time your alarm goes off.
- **Stay away from stimulants like caffeine.** Avoid stimulants in the evening, including chocolate, caffeinated sodas, coffee and teas. They will delay sleep and increase arousal during the night.
- **Avoid bright light around the house before bed.** Use dimmer switches in the living room, bathroom and bedroom before bed. If you read in bed, do so by a small wattage bulb.
- **Keep the bed for rest, relaxation and sleeping.** Avoid watching TV or using your laptop computer in bed. If you read, avoid material that is upsetting or stimulating and read by a dim light.
- **Avoid exercise near bedtime.** Avoid exercise for 2-3 hours before bed. However, using gentle yoga with mindful, slow breathing may evoke a sense of relaxation and winding down that may help with sleep.
- **Don't go to bed hungry.** Avoid heavy meals right before bed; however, you may have a light healthy snack like yogurt, a handful of nuts, or a piece of fruit.
- **Keep bedtime routines.** Keep routines on your normal schedule. A cup of herbal tea an hour before bed can begin a routine.
- **Avoid looking at the clock.** If you wake up in the middle of the night, don't look at the clock. Watching the time in the middle of the night can cause anxiety and contribute to sleeplessness.
- **Practice slow, deep breathing.** If you have trouble falling asleep or wake up in the

middle of the night, try 5-10 minutes of slow, deep belly breathing, shifting all of your attention to watching your breath.

- **Use the 30 minute rule:** If you can't get to sleep for over 30 minutes, and have tried slow, deep breathing, get out of bed and do something boring in dim light until you are sleepy.
- **Mask noisy surroundings:** Use a fan or a white noise generator to create a constant background sound.
- **Recognize the price of a "night cap."** Alcohol may help you get to sleep, but it will cause you to wake up throughout the night. It is worse if you have sleep apnea. Snoring may also become worse with alcohol.
- **Get feedback:** If you have a sleeping partner, ask them if they notice any snoring, leg movements and/or pauses in breathing. You may have a sleep disorder. Take your concerns to your doctor.
- **Don't stress!** If you feel you are not getting enough sleep, worrying only makes matters worse. Try the suggestions above and know you will sleep eventually.

A P P E N D I X   D
~ Emotional Self-Health and Sacral Chakra ~

Journal Writing for Emotional Self-Health

1. Identify an emotional reaction. _____

2. Label the specific emotion. _____

3. Close your eyes and **FEEL** *the emotion*. Where do you feel the emotion in your body? What does it feel like?

4. Open your eyes and write. *I feel...*

5. Describe the situation.

6. What other situation does this remind you of and why?

7. Share this conscious remembrance with another person.

8. Release this emotion through a ritual, a scream, a shout, forgiveness, a verbal affirmation, or a body movement.

9. Notice how you feel NOW.

A P P E N D I X E
~ Emotional Self-Health and Sacral Chakra ~

Suggestions for Enhancing Intimacy and Sex

Set the stage for good communication
- Turn off the TV and telephone, and schedule a time when you are not exhausted and are free from interruption.
- Speak from your own feelings: "I feel," not "You make me feel," or "Everyone knows..." Use "I" statements that speak from the heart. "I feel... I believe..."
- Allow each other equal time to share.
- Make eye contact and listen respectfully.
- Make a specific time to continue your discussion if you feel it is not completed.

Write an Ad for a Lover Who Touches Your Heart and Soul
This is a fun opportunity to express your fantasies and dreams to each other for all you wish in an intimate partner. Give yourself 10-15 minutes to compose the personal ad. Let yourself be soulful, sexy, inventive, funny and as specific as you can be.
- Begin by writing WANTED; and then let your imagination run wild about what you want.
- Then write, IN TURN FOR WHICH, and be specific about what you would like to offer your ideal lover in the best of all possible worlds.
- When you are finished, read them aloud to each other.

Write a "Letter to My Lover"
Partners can write this directly to each other
- Begin with the positive—what you truly love about your partner and something you feel works really well for the two of you.
- The rest of the letter can focus on something your want your partner to understand about you—your wants, needs, fears, wishes for contact, communication and meaning.

Touching Closed Eye Meditation

This is a great way to communicate and connect without words. The intention is to keep your eyes closed and not talk. Just see where it leads you, or where you lead each other.

- Begin by sitting facing each other with knees touching, wearing loose comfortable clothing or lingerie.
- Set a timer for 10-15 minutes.
- Close your eyes and touch foreheads (third eye) .
- Focus on your breathing, sensing your own breath and your partner's breath.
- You may want to lightly place a hand on your partner's heart center and one on the sacral center.
- Follow your intuition and senses until the timer goes off. Do whatever comes naturally.

Practice Sacred Sexuality

Buy a book or a video that shares ideas related to Tantra and the ancient spiritual practices of sexuality.

A P P E N D I X   F
~ Occupational Self-Health and Solar Plexus Chakra ~

Balancing Values in Work and Well-Being

Personal Values: Circle all of the values that have meaning and importance to you.
Work Environment: Circle all of those that your work environment or daily tasks provide and support.

Personal Values	**Work Environment**
Autonomy	Autonomy
Community	Community
Self-expression	Self-expression
Creativity	Creativity
Money	Money
Recognition	Recognition
Contribution	Contribution
Leadership	Leadership
Authority	Authority
Responsibility	Responsibility
Enjoyment	Enjoyment
Spirituality	Spirituality
Accomplishment	Accomplishment
Relationships	Relationships
Friendships	Friendships
Honesty	Honesty
Communication	Communication
Integrity	Integrity
Continuous Learning	Continuous Learning
Teaching	Teaching
Personal growth	Personal growth
Attaining goals	Attaining goals
Security	Security
Appreciation	Appreciation
Humor	Humor
Harmony	Harmony
Variety	Variety
Challenge	Challenge

Intentions for change and enhancing Occupational Self-Health: Where are the mis-matches?

If there are personal values that are not currently supported by work or other activity choices, list those values with 2-3 ideas for creating opportunities to express those values.

157

A P P E N D I X   G
~ Occupational Self-Health and Solar Plexus Chakra ~

Canvas of Personal Power

Draw an outline of both hands on this sheet of paper or a blank sheet of paper. It's okay if they over lap, just make sure all fingertips are visible. On each fingertip, write something you have accomplished, you feel good about doing, or are skilled at doing. Then fill the paper with spontaneous thoughts and statements beginning with "I CAN…"

WORKSHEET
Canvas of Personal Power

A P P E N D I X   H
~ Relational Self-Health and Heart Chakra ~

Healing Pathways Meditation

Begin by lying or sitting in a comfortable position. Breathe in deeply and slowly, following each breath, in…and out. Notice the breathing for a moment, quietly, without judging or trying to change your breath.

Now bring your attention to your heart center. See this center of your body as a rich, warm color of green. With each inhale, breathe in unconditional love into your heart center. Fill your heart with unconditional love. Feel the love expanding with each breath. Now, with each exhale, breathe out unconditional love, feeling that love gently move out from you, back into you, out from you. Feel the gentle yet powerful cycle of love, giving and receiving love.

Now with your awareness on your heart, so filled with love, allow the flow of this love from your heart to move down the right side of your body to the base of the spine, carrying your heart energy to your base chakra. Fuel your sense of grounding, belonging, safety and stability with the energy of love. Visualize the color red, expanding with each breath, at the base of your spine. Send all of the strength, safety and grounding energy from your base chakra up the left side of your body to the heart. Your heart is open to receive this energy.

Now, allow your heart energy—the love—to move up the right side of your body to your throat. Carry love to your throat chakra, pulsating in the color blue. Allow the love from your heart to expand and strengthen your voice, your will, your ability to express clearly your wants, desires, needs and creativity. See the color blue in your throat expanding with each breath, and with your next exhale send all of your beautiful self-expression down the left side of your body, back into the center of your heart. Feel the fullness of your heart.

With your next exhale, allow this full, expansive heart energy to move down the right side of your body to your sacral chakra, your lower belly and lower back. See the vibrant, passionate color of orange fill the space of your sacral chakra, fueling your sense of desire, sensuality, sexuality, pleasure, passion, authentic emotional expression and connection with others. See the color orange expanding, with each breath. With the next exhale allow the pleasure, self-nurturance and passion from your sacral chakra to travel up the left side of the body into the center of the heart, the heart breathing in and generously receiving the pleasure of this energy.

As the heart's fullness continues to expand, allow the powerful energy of love to move up the right side of the body to your third eye chakra, the center of your brow. As you feel the color indigo expanding in your third eye, be aware of your innate wisdom, your intuition, your openness to learning and expanding. See this indigo and your third eye expanding, pulsating, vibrating with energy. With your next exhale, send the expansiveness of your wisdom down the left side of your body, integrating this energy into the heart, filling the heart with your innate knowingness. Feel the fullness of the heart, the love and truth expanding and deepening.

With your next exhale, allow this love and truth to flow freely down the right side of the body to your solar plexus, the center of your belly, your chakra of personal power, self-esteem, self-confidence and responsibility. See the brilliant, bright and fiery color of yellow expanding in this center. Feel the warmth, the radiance, the strength and the personal honor. As this color yellow expands with each breath, allow it to radiate, brighter and brighter, feeling the radiance of your unique and powerful SELF. Now with the next exhale, guide this radiance up the left side of your body, bringing this personal radiance and light into the heart, the love in the heart continuing to expand with each breath.

Continue to feel this expanded heart energy, radiant, strong, passionate, creative and wise. See this energy move up the right side of the body to the crown of the head, or slightly above the crown of the head, fueling the brilliance of the color violet, your crown chakra. As this violet color expands, feel your connection to all there is, your sense of purpose and your feelings of inspiration expand outside of your physical body. Experience your essence glowing. With your next exhale, allow this essence to move and flow gently down the left side of the body, into the heart center that is now pulsating with a rainbow of colors and a richness of sensations.

As you continue to breathe, slowly, rhythmically, feel the heart center move into a place of peace, centeredness, and quiet calm. Trusting the body's inherent wisdom, feel the smooth flow of energy from the toes to the crown of the head to the finger tips. Notice, witness and TRUST. Love is the power and the heart is the center. Allow its fullness to radiate healing pulses of light and bliss throughout every cell of your body.

Before opening your eyes express gratitude to your heart for its knowingness, its gentleness, its capacity for love and healing. Take two or three deep cleansing breaths and slowly open your eyes.

Visualization for Healing Pathways Meditation

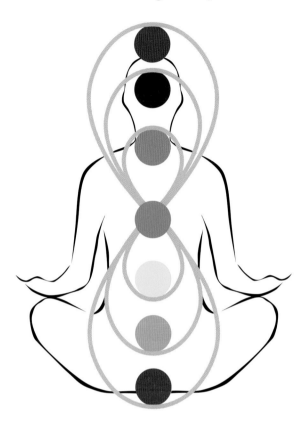

A P P E N D I X I
~ Self-Expressional Self-Health and Throat Chakra ~

The Art of Communication

- **Seek first to understand.** Try putting yourself in the other person's shoes.
- **Listen and look intently.** Maintain eye contact and body language that says "I'm listening."
- **Speak clearly from the heart.** Use words such as "I believe," "I feel," "I need or I want."
- **Open your ears and your mind.** Let go of preconceived notions or judgments.
- **Practice dialogue, not debate.** Let go of the need to be right. Practice non-judgmental acceptance.

Keys to Plain Talk
- Ask yourself what you want, from your heart.
- Ask yourself what you need.
- Ask yourself how you feel (anger is often a mask for fear or hurt).
- Sketch a verbal plan to help you communicate with others to achieve your objectives.
- Use words that unite (we, us, our).
- Beware of setting I against YOU.
- Focus on how what you want will benefit the other person.
- Avoid defining a winner or a loser.
- Use language that emphasizes potential rather than limiting it.

Communicate Using "I" messages

I feel _____ **when** _____ **because** _____.
I need *or* **I would like**_____.

Become a Better Listener
- Practice creative self-restraint.

- Give feedback that you are intently listening: nod, smile, react.
- Use verbal mirrors. **Repeat, "echo" or rephrase** key phrases to let the other person know you are hearing and understanding.
- Tell the other person you understand.
- Don't neglect your response, but suspend it long enough to hear out the other person.
- Listen so you can focus on the other person's needs.
- Stay with the main thought.
- Develop what interests you and find common ground.

A P P E N D I X   J
~ Mental Self-Health and Third Eye Chakra ~

A Guide for Visualization

Visualization is the technique of using your mind through imagination to create what you want in life. Imagination is the ability to create an idea or mental picture in your mind. Focused visualization allows you to use your imagination to create a clear image of some thing or situation you wish to manifest in your life.

Read through each set of instructions as many times as necessary to guide yourself through the visualization process. Start with *visualizing a memory* so you can quickly and easily experience the power of the mind to create a present reality.

General Guidelines
• Practice visualization daily. It is most effective following meditation, when your mind is clear and your body is relaxed.
• Find a quiet place, free from distractions.
• Relax your mind and body. Take three or four deep breaths. Breathe in through your nose, out through your mouth, expand your abdomen with each breath.
• Close your eyes and picture a large blank movie screen.

Visualizing a Memory
• Bring to mind a picture on the movie screen of one of your favorite memories (a vacation, time with friends or family, a favorite place or activity).
• Place yourself in that place and time. Picture in your mind:
  - how you got there (walk, ride, run).
  - what you are wearing (type of clothing, colors).
  - the people with you (family, friends, strangers).
  - your surroundings (outside, inside, temperature, weather, objects, nature).
  - any particular odors or aromas that surround you (water, smoke, baking).
  - what you are doing (imagine your body moving, assuming positions).
• Think about what you like best about this memory and why.

Visualizing an Intention

- Picture yourself experiencing the situation you wish to manifest.
- Use your imagination to place yourself in that particular environment
- Clearly picture your surroundings, including sights, smells, temperature, people, sounds that support your desired situation.
- Clearly see yourself in the situation as strong, confident, joyous, calm, content and successful. Watch yourself accept into your life the situation or intention your have manifested with grace and peace.
- Notice the people around you as loving and supportive in your manifestation.

A P P E N D I X   K
~ Mental Self-Health and Third Eye Chakra ~

Color Exercise

Take a blank piece of paper (or use the next page), pencil and markers or paint. Draw three 2-inch diameter circles.

1) Close your eyes and feel a color that soothes and relaxes you. Paint or color this color in the first circle.

2) Now close your eyes. Imagine you have just heard some exciting news. You feel joyful and happy! What color do you see that expresses that feeling? Paint this color in the second circle.

3) Now close your eyes and feel a color that is uncomfortable, rough, or irritating to you. Now paint this color with jagged, uneven lines in or around the third circle.

Take some time to notice how you work with or integrate these colors in your life. Have you used them for painting or decorating a room? Do you dress in the "joy" colors when you need a lift? Do you know a space that is painted in the "yucky" color that you avoid or feel uncomfortable in?

Make conscious choices to include the colors in your life that "feed" you positively.

WORKSHEET
Color Exercise

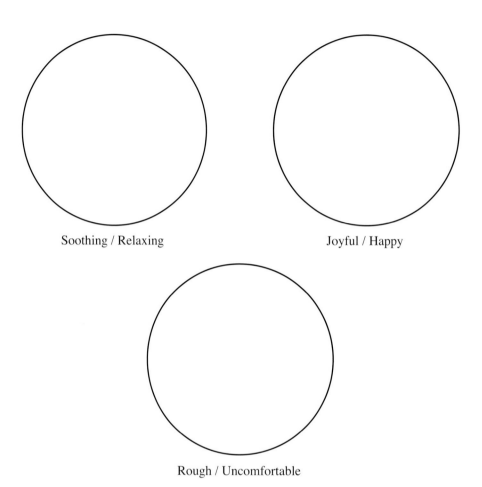

Soothing / Relaxing   Joyful / Happy

Rough / Uncomfortable

A P P E N D I X   L
~ Mental Self-Health and Third Eye Chakra ~

Examine Limiting Core Beliefs

Take a moment to review the following core beliefs related to each chakra or energy center. Mark any statement that rings true for you. Then take a few moments to reflect on how that belief shows up and influences your every day life.

Trust/Base Chakra:
- ☐ I don't believe there is a benevolent universe.
- ☐ I can't let go and/or don't know how to trust.
- ☐ I can't give up control to something larger than myself.
- ☐ I will be taken advantage of if I don't constantly look out for myself.

Flow/Sacral Chakra:
- ☐ Unexpected changes overwhelm me. I won't know what to do.
- ☐ I need to have security to feel safe in my life.
- ☐ I am afraid change will hurt me.
- ☐ Change is too difficult and painful. I would rather keep things the same.

Self-Esteem and Responsibility/Solar Plexus Chakra:
- ☐ I am a victim to forces beyond my control.
- ☐ I don't have the power to change my life.
- ☐ I don't know how to deal with difficult situations.
- ☐ I am not good enough to be successful.
- ☐ I am afraid of stepping into my own power.

Love and Relationships/Heart Chakra:
- ☐ I am not loveable or worthy of love.
- ☐ Loving others is more important that loving myself.
- ☐ It is more important to give than to receive.

THE ART OF SELF-HEALTH

□ Seeking support from others is a sign of weakness.

□ Other people don't have time to give me support or help.

Personal Expression/Throat Chakra:

□ I don't deserve health, wealth and abundance.

□ Asking for what I want is selfish.

□ I'm never sure what I want and need.

□ Being honest with others will hurt their feelings.

□ I don't know how to create or be creative.

Positive Attitude/Third Eye Chakra:

□ Life is a struggle.

□ I can't change my body (this illness/disease). Nothing I do makes a difference.

□ I am a victim of circumstances beyond my control.

□ If I break the rules I'll be punished.

□ I can't change the way I think or what I think.

Connection/Crown Chakra:

□ I am all alone in my life.

□ It is impossible and impractical to have feelings of peace and joy all of the time.

□ I don't know how to connect with divine guidance and intelligence.

□ My situation is completely different than anyone else's.

Limiting Belief Turnaround with New Intentions for Self-Health

> **State your issue.** Ask yourself: Where do I feel stuck or contracted? If possible, state it as a limiting belief.

Example: *"I can't seem to find time to incorporate a walk into my schedule everyday."*

Limiting Belief: "I am a victim of circumstances (time demands) beyond my control."

My issue/limiting belief: _____

> **Create a turnaround statement.** Ask yourself: What do I
> want? How would I like it to be?

Example: *"I want to find time 30 minutes a day to walk or exercise."*

Refine the turnaround into an intention. An intention is making a positive, first-person, succinct, specific statement as if it were true.

Example: *"I am fully capable and responsible for managing my daily time, and able to create 30 minutes each day for walking or exercise."*

My turnaround statement: _____

_____

My intention: _____

_____

> **Check the believability of your intention.** Ask yourself:
> Do I believe this is possible? Adjust your intention as needed.

Example: Do you need to revise the time factor to 15 minutes instead of 30 minutes?

My revision to my intention for full believability: _____

_____

> **Embody your intention.** Use visualization, physical activity,
> spiritual practice or pictures to engrain the intention into your
> system. See it and feel it as though it already exists.

A P P E N D I X   M
~ Spiritual Self-Health and Crown Chakra ~

Gratitude

Studies show that the daily practice of gratitude results in higher levels of alertness, enthusiasm, determination, optimism and energy. People who express gratitude regularly experience more reciprocal love and kindness and less depression and stress. Gratitude is life-empowering! Gratitude promotes health for mind, body and spirit.

- **Gratitude is a choice.** Focus on things that are good and right in your life as opposed to things that are not.
- **Gratitude is conscious awareness.** Recognize all the abundance there is for us in life and acknowledge the gift.
- **Gratitude focus acts like a magnet.** When you focus on those things you are most grateful for, you give those aspects of your life more power. Your world is more full and alive!

Ways to Practice Gratitude

- Set aside quiet reflection time. Examine your day and seek out all that you are grateful for. Move beyond material blessings and focus on relationships, the beauty of nature, music that fills your soul and challenges that have made you stronger.

- Use a journal to express your gratitude. Writing can bring things to the surface and provide a private, non-judgmental listener.

- Take a walk and focus on the trees, colors, textures, sounds and earthy smells.

- Take time to focus on the health and vitality of your body with gratitude. Slowly scan your body and thank each part (legs, arms, heart, lungs, eyes, etc.) for supporting your ability to live and interact at this time.

- Express gratitude to your self for the special gifts and talents you have and the ability to be of service to others.

- Show appreciation to other people by writing a note or sending a card expressing your gratitude for their presence in your life. This brings joy to you and them!

- Notice how you *feel* when you are in a state of gratitude — full, calm, warm, inviting, loving, generous. More gratitude, more good feelings!

A P P E N D I X   N
~ Spiritual Self-Health and Crown Chakra ~

A Guide for Mindfulness Meditation

While many meditation techniques may be more easily learned with an experienced guide, mindfulness meditation can certainly be self-taught and positively experienced with practice. Meditation allows you to experience a state of restful alertness, which assists physical and mental relaxation while improving mental clarity. Read through these instructions as many times as needed to feel comfortable with the process and allow yourself several sessions of practice to become comfortable and familiar with both process and experience.

General Guidelines
- Schedule and practice meditation daily for a minimum of 10 minutes per session.
- Find a comfortable place free from distractions.
- Release all expectations you may have about the experience.
- Allow yourself to BE.

Mindfulness Meditation Process

- Sit comfortably in a chair or on the floor. Close your eyes.

- Allow your jaw to become loose and slack, with your lips slightly parted.

- Begin by taking three slow, deep breaths. Breathe in through your nose and out through your nose or slightly open mouth, expanding your abdomen with each breath.

- Allow your breathing to return to a normal rate.

- Become an observer of your breath. Visualize the air moving in and out of your lungs. Note the rate and depth of your breathing. Do not try to adjust your breathing. SIMPLY

OBSERVE the breath.

- As thoughts, feelings, images or sounds in your surroundings appear, simply let them float through your mind. Allow the thoughts to go through your mind without expressing positive or negative feelings about them.

- Look for and stay in the "gap" between thoughts.

- If at any time you find it difficult to let go of a thought, feeling or image, simply shift your focus back to observing your breath. IN.......and.......OUT.

- Continue this exercise for 10-30 minutes.

- Prior to opening your eyes, take 2-3 slow, deep breaths.

- Open your eyes and sit quietly for a few minutes. Note how you feel and any other sensations you may have (warmth, tingling, relaxation, etc.).

- You may note or remember moments of thinking "nothing" or "slipping into the gap between thoughts." This is common, enjoyable and part of the process.

NOTE: Focus on the breath can be replaced with a word or sound (mantra). Experiment with the technique that is most comfortable for you. Examples of mantras include: "peace," "I am calm," "Om," "Ah," "I am."

A P P E N D I X   O

Moving Chakra Charger

Use the following visualizations while doing any kind of repetitive exercise or movement, such as walking, running, riding a bike, swimming, dancing, using an elliptical or stair step piece of equipment. This is a great way to be present in your body while moving and consciously focusing energy into each chakra. Feel free to add your own variations and trust your inner guidance in your visualization.

- Focus on your feet and legs. Feel the toes, feet, ankles and legs as they move and come in contact with the earth. Visualize a deep red color moving into your lower body and the exchange of that color with the earth as you move. Imagine drawing in sensations of strength, stability, trust and belonging.

- Focus on your hips and pelvis. Bring the sensation and quality of water into this area of your body, allowing an easy flow and movement of your hips. Visualize a vibrant orange color in waves of sensuous rhythm washing through your hips and pelvis.

- Focus on your solar plexus, your mid-belly. Imagine a bright yellow light radiating from the center of your belly. Feel the largeness and confidence of your presence. As you move, do so with power, strength and confidence. Imagine the fire of this bright yellow light, burning away any challenge or obstacle in your way.

- Focus on your heart center. If you are able, open your arms like wings and give your heart free flight. Imagine a rich color of green spreading from your heart and into your arms. Pay attention to your breathing. With each breath in, draw in unconditional and nurturing self-love. With each breath out, send that love into the world.

- Focus on your throat and neck. Feel the subtle vibration in this area as your breath moves in and out. Imagine a clear, blue color in this area of your body and with every exhale imagine only your truth and creativity being expressed. If you can, say out loud

"YES" with each exhale…yes, to living a full, meaningful life today.

- Focus on your third eye. While you have already been exercising this chakra, now visualize a deep indigo blue field or screen ahead of you. On this screen, see yourself as healthy, vital and peaceful. With each step or movement, imagine "stepping into" this self and merging completely, becoming exactly what you see.

- Focus on the crown of your head. Imagine a soft violet light bathing your entire body. With each breath, this light expands out, merging with your surroundings. You are becoming connected to everything around you. There is no separation. As you breathe in, you breathe in the same air that supports the trees. As you breathe out, you share a part of your self with every other living thing.

179

APPENDIX P
~ Tools for Self-Health Reference Chart ~

The following chart can serve as a guide for selecting and applying simple self-health tools for each of the seven dimensions of self-health. It is by no means all-inclusive, and is meant to serve only as a general guide.

	Physical **Base Chakra**	Emotional **Sacral Chakra**	Occupational **Solar Plexus Chakra**	Relational **Heart Chakra**	Self-Expressional **Throat Chakra**	Mental **Third Eye Chakra**	Spiritual **Crown Chakra**
Deep Breathing	x	x	x	x	x	x	x
Relaxation	x	x	x	x	x	x	
Sleep	x	x	x	x	x	x	x
Journal Writing	x	x	x	x	x	x	
Yoga	x	x	x	x	x	x	x
The Nia Technique®	x	x	x	x	x	x	x
Pilates	x		x			x	
Tai Chi	x	x	x			x	x
Walking, Cycling, Running, Swimming, Dancing	x	x	x	x	x	x	x
Healthful Nutrition	x	x	x	x	x	x	
Laughter	x	x	x	x	x	x	x
Sacred Sex	x	x		x	x	x	x
Creative Activities, Play, Games	x	x	x	x	x	x	
Singing, Chanting, Toning, Listening to Music	x	x			x	x	
Meditation	x	x	x	x	x	x	x
Visualization/Imagery	x	x	x	x	x	x	x
Color Therapy	x	x	x		x	x	x
Gratitude	x	x	x	x	x	x	x
Nature Walks	x			x		x	x
Speaking from your Heart, Listening	x	x	x	x	x	x	
Aromatherapy	x	x				x	x
Music Therapy	x	x		x	x	x	x
Loving family & friendships	x	x		x	x		x
Pets	x	x		x	x	x	x

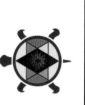

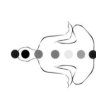

APPENDIX Q
The Chakras and The Art of Self-Health

CHAKRA	In Balance	Out of Balance	Self-Health Remedies
1 *Physical Self-Health* **Base/Red** Element: Earth	• Grounded • Feelings of safety and security • Basic trust and feelings of belonging • Strong immune system • Good health, vitality and energy	• Fear about safety and security • Weight problems • Frequent illness • Sluggish, listless and tired • Problems with feet, knees, hips and/or base of spine • Sciatica • Immune related disorders	• Seek support (family, friends, community) • Deep breathing • Pleasurable movement • Tasteful, balanced nutrition • Conscious relaxation and adequate sleep • Create beauty and comfort in your home
2 *Emotional Self-Health* **Sacral/Orange** Element: Water	• Ability to experience pleasure • Healthy and authentic emotional expression • Ability to adapt and change • Nurturing of self and others • Graceful movement	• Rigidity of body and attitudes • Controlling beliefs and attitudes • Fear of change • Denial or excess of pleasure, sex, emotions and attachments • Loss of appetite/ and passion for food, sex, life • Disorders of reproductive system, urinary system, low back	• Acknowledge desires and express emotions • Be honest with self and others • Self-nurturance • Healthy boundaries in relationships • Pleasurable or expressive body movement • Bathing • Embrace change and let go • Healthy, sacred sexuality
3 *Occupational Self-Health* **Solar Plexus/Yellow** Element: Fire	• Confident • Responsible and reliable • Warm personality • Spontaneous and playful • Sense of one's personal power • Individuation • Good self-esteem	• Low self-esteem • Unreliable and irresponsible • Stubborn • Competitive • Dominating and controlling • Dependent • Eating disorders • Diabetes • Low energy and chronic fatigue	• Acknowledge unique gifts and talents • Break inertia and move powerfully • Find meaning in all you do • Take responsibility for your SELF • Identify and claim your personal power • Strengthen your core muscles

	Healthy	Imbalanced	Practices
4 ***Relational Self-Health*** **Heart/Green** Element: Air	• Self-Loving • Easily love others • Compassionate and empathetic • Altruistic • Peaceful • Forgiving • Open hearted • Joyous	• Resentful and intolerant • Self-loathing • Anti-social and withdrawn • Jealous • Co-dependent • Lack of empathy and compassion • Unforgiving • Fear of intimacy • Disorders of lungs, breasts, heart and arms • Sunken chest • Tension between shoulder blades	• Consciously open your heart • Practice SELF love, understanding and compassion • Practice forgiveness and let go of resentment • Listen to your heart • Nurture "energy-giving" relationships • Give and receive loving touch
5 ***Self-Expressional Self-Health*** **Throat/Light Blue** Element: Sound	• Clear, resonant voice • Good listener • Creative expression and living • Clear, open communication • Good sense of timing and rhythm • Positive language and self talk • Express needs, desires and will	• Introversion and shyness • Poor listening and too much talking • Fear of speaking • Fear of trying something new or creative • Small, weak voice • Poor rhythm • Disorders of throat, thyroid, ears, neck and voice • Tightness of jaw, clenched teeth	• Always speak your truth • Practice singing and toning • Practice creativity • Practice silence and listening • Practice positive self-talk • Journal writing • Listen to beautiful music
6 ***Mental Self-Health*** **Third Eye/Indigo** Element: Light	• Intuitive • Imaginative • Able to focus and concentrate • Able to visualize • Perceptive • Good memory • Able to access and remember dreams	• Poor memory • Lack of imagination • Difficulty focusing or concentrating • "Tunnel" vision • Inability to remember dreams • Headaches • Vision problems	• Witness your thoughts • Practice visualization • Re-visit pleasant memories • Practice present moment awareness • Examine your beliefs • Change your mind • Use color to enliven or calm
7 ***Spiritual Self-Health*** **Crown/Violet** Element: Thought	• Open minded • Thoughtful • Aware • Broad understanding • Wisdom • Sense of spiritual connection • Able to see the larger pattern • Able to question • Trust "not knowing"	• Rigid belief systems • Spiritual cynicism • Difficulty learning • Apathy • Hopelessness • Confusion • Over intellectualization • Disassociation from the body • Brain disorders • Migraines	• Meditation • Silence • Prayer • Connect with nature • Be open minded • Continue to learn • Practice gratitude everyday

A C K N O W L E D G M E N T S

I don't know if you can thank your own soul, but I do thank mine for the quiet whispers, subtle wake up calls and the strong nudges to stay awake and conscious through each life changing and expanding process. Most importantly, I am grateful for the accompaniment of those soul companions along the way who have witnessed, unconditionally loved, supported, questioned, laughed and cried with me. These are the friends and family who encouraged me to let go when I needed to and hang on tight for the ride when I needed to.

An incredible, special group of people volunteered to review the concept and content of this book, graciously giving feedback and guidance along the way. I am grateful to these men and women for sharing their hearts, souls, minds and self-health experiences with me and the pages of this book. Heartfelt gratitude to Teresa Brimacombe, Collette Jandura-Buzzard, Winnie Dunn, Joan Jarrett, Beth LaRue, Bill LaRue, Mindie Pearcy, George Satterlee, Barb Unell and Joan Vermaire.

Special gratitude goes to my loving partner Bill LaRue, not only for his unwavering support, but also for sharing his talent and passion for photography in taking the pictures for the book. Thanks also to the friends of Lendonwood Gardens in Grove, Oklahoma for providing some of the best that nature offers as a back drop for photos. My loving thanks to Janice LaRue who provided valuable format and editing guidance, and to Pamela Hawkins a talented and wonderful graphic artist for the design of the book, cover and illustrations.

As my first and longest lived teachers, I am eternally grateful to my parents, Vernon and Mary Frantz, who somehow instilled within me the power of my "anything is possible" mindset. Their love both fueled and allowed for my self-discoveries by sticking my neck out and occasionally exploring the edges in life.

There are many others who have shared this journey with me, serving as sounding boards, providing resources, reviewing selected excerpts and simply offering encouragement and support toward completion of the process. These precious friends and colleagues include Valerie Campbell, Toby Evans, Megan Hill, Amie Jew, MD, Christian Lett, Gretchen Grace Lindsay, Suzanne Lovell, Jane Murray, MD, Carol Rydell, Doreen Shea, Colleen Trimble and Lisa Whitlow.

BIBLIOGRAPHY

Anatomy of Spirit, Caroline Myss; Harmony Books

You Can Heal Your Life, Louise Hay; Hay House, Inc.

Frontiers of Health, Christine Page M.D.; Rider

Eastern Body Western Mind, Anodea Judith; Celestial Arts

Wheels of Life, Anodea Judith; Llewellyn Publications

Molecules of Emotions, Candace B. Pert, Ph.D.; Touchstone

The Power of Now, Eckhart Tolle; New World Library

The Nia Technique Brown Belt Manual, Debbie and Carlos Rosas; The Nia Technique

The Triple Goddess Tarot, Isha Lerner; Bear and Company

The Pleasure Prescription, Paul Pearsall, Ph.D.; Hunter House

The Power of Intention, Dr. Wayne W. Dyer; Hay House, Inc.

What the Bleep Do We Know!?; William Arntz, Betsy Chasse, Mark Vicente;
 Health Communications Inc.

Awakening and Healing the Rainbow Body, Jessie E. Ayani; Heart of the Sun

Wisdom from The Mastery of Love, Don Miguel Ruiz; Peter Pauper Press, Inc.

The Four Agreements, Don Miguel Ruiz; Amber-Allen Publishing

Spiritual Alchemy, Christine Page, M.D.; Rider

A New Earth, Eckhart Tolle; A Plume Book, Penguin Group

Natural Health, Natural Medicine, Andrew Weil, M.D.; Houghton Mifflin Company

Women's Bodies, Women's Wisdom, Christiane Northrup, M.D.; Bantam Books

The Untethered Soul, Michael A. Singer; New Harbinger Publications, Inc.

The Divine Matrix, Gregg Braden; Hay House, Inc.

Animal Speak, Ted Andrews; Llewellyn Publications

ABOUT THE AUTHOR

Carol F. LaRue, is a licensed occupational therapist, a brown belt certified Nia Technique® movement instructor, certified Pilates mat exercise instructor, a certified instructor of Transformation Meditation and certified teacher of The Art of Feminine Presence™. She is the creator of specialized movement and support classes for women cancer survivors "Moving into Wellness™" and "Restorative Balanced Moves™." Carol loves sharing tools and practices that help people feel better and enjoy life with more energy, effectiveness and meaning, and is available for speaking engagements, workshops and private coaching. Carol joyfully brings a sense of grounded, "real life practicality" into all of her teachings.

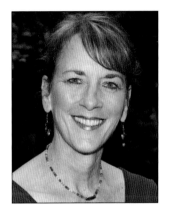

She lives on Grand Lake in Oklahoma with her husband Bill and their sweet dog Dottie.

Carol may be contacted by e-mail at: carol@artofselfhealth.com or by phone at 913.341.6607.

RESOURCES

Carol schedules and hosts private and semi-private Self-Health retreats at Turtlecove Treehouse on Grand Lake O' the Cherokees near Grove, Oklahoma. Visit www.turtlecovetreehouse.com for more information.

Guests are able to "start where they are" by customizing their retreat with a varied menu of personal coaching services and individualized support that includes:

- Integrative Wellness Coaching (Art of Self-Health model)
- Personal Movement Coaching
- Mindfulness Meditation Training
- Art of Feminine Presence™ Coaching

Visit www.artofselfhealth.com for more information.